FACT AND FICTION OF HEALTHY VISION

Recent Titles in
The Praeger Series on Contemporary Health and Living

A Guide to Getting the Best Health Care for Your Child
Roy Benaroch, M.D.

Defending and Parenting Children Who Learn Differently: Lessons from Edison's
Mother
Scott Teel

Ordinary Miracles: Learning from Breast Cancer Survivors
S. David Nathanson, M.D.

FACT AND FICTION OF HEALTHY VISION

Eye Care for Adults and Children

Clyde K. Kitchen

The Praeger Series on Contemporary Health and Living
Julie Silver, Series Editor

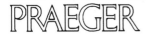

Westport, Connecticut
London

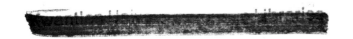

Library of Congress Cataloging-in-Publication Data

Kitchen, Clyde K., 1933–
Fact and fiction of healthy vision : eye care for adults and children / Clyde K. Kitchen.
  p. cm. – (The Praeger series on contemporary health and living ; ISSN 1932–8079)
  Includes bibliographical references and index.
  ISBN 978–0–275–99345–0 (alk. paper)
  1. Eye—Care and hygiene. 2. Vision. I. Title.
 RE51.K5887 2007
 617.7–dc22 2007006831

British Library Cataloguing in Publication Data is available.

Library of Congress Catalog Card Number: 2007006831
ISBN-13: 978–0–275–99345–0
ISBN-10: 0–275–99345–0
ISSN: 1932–8079

First published in 2007

Praeger Publishers, 88 Post Road West, Westport, CT 06881
An imprint of Greenwood Publishing Group, Inc.
www.praeger.com

Printed in the United States of America

The paper used in this book complies with the
Permanent Paper Standard issued by the National
Information Standards Organization (Z39.48–1984).

10 9 8 7 6 5 4 3 2 1

This book is for general information only. No book can ever substitute for the judgment of a
medical professional. If you have worries or concerns, contact your doctor.

Some of the names and details of individuals discussed in this book have been changed to protect
the patients' identities. Some of the stories may be composites of patient interactions created for
illustrative purposes.

CONTENTS

Series Foreword

Over the past hundred years, there have been incredible medical break-throughs that have prevented or cured illness in billions of people and helped many more improve their health while living with chronic conditions. A few of the most important twentieth-century discoveries include antibiotics, organ transplants, and vaccines. The twenty-first century has already heralded important new treatments including such things as a vaccine to prevent human papillomavirus from infecting and potentially leading to cervical cancer in women. Polio is on the verge of being eradicated worldwide, making it only the second infectious disease behind smallpox to ever be erased as a human health threat.

In this series, experts from many disciplines share with readers important and updated medical knowledge. All aspects of health are considered including subjects that are disease-specific and preventive medical care. Disseminating this information will help individuals to improve their health as well as researchers to determine where there are gaps in our current knowledge and policy-makers to assess the most pressing needs in health care.

Series Editor Julie Silver, M.D.
Assistant Professor
Harvard Medical School
Department of Physical Medicine and Rehabiliation

ACKNOWLEDGMENTS

I would like to acknowledge the help of Dr. Julie Silver, my Series Editor, and Debbie Carvalko, my Acquisitions Editor, who made what seemed like unscalable barriers become more like minor hurdles, something I can handle.

Also, I would like to show appreciation for my ophthalmology training at the University of Iowa, under the tutelage of professors Dr. A.E. Braley, Dr. Fred Blodi, Dr. P.J. Leinfelder, Dr. Herman Burian, Dr. Robert Watzke, and Dr. Mansour Armaly.

Inspirational leadership has been displayed by Dr. Gunter von Noorden, Dr. Richard Schultz, Dr. Melvin Rubin, Dr. John Lynn, and Dr. Bruce Spivey, all friends of mine in residency training at the University of Iowa, and who entered academics while I went into private practice.

I am especially grateful to my wife Janet, whose encouragement and support made this book possible. Not to be forgotten, I feel privileged to have many wonderful patients who have inspired me to put on paper some of the things we have talked about over the past several years.

Introduction

Every day, comments are made in newsprint, and on radio or television about eye care, from promotional pitches to descriptions of new discoveries. An eye surgeon advertises his services, often in multiple offices, as a specialist in correcting nearsightedness, farsightedness, astigmatism, cataracts, presbyopia, and keratoconus. I wonder how many people know what these conditions are and why surgery would be involved. Over the radio, there are statements about someone, frequently the newsman himself who had been legally blind and was made able to see 20/20 after getting his eyes fixed by laser. A lady says she signed up for eye exercises advertised on radio and was able to stop wearing her glasses, which were making her eyes weak. Another advertisement states that special over-the-counter eye drops can reduce symptoms of cataract. A well-known radio newsman reports that a lady who used the vitamins he promotes was able to regain her vision. Then a tennis buddy asks me about his ninety-four-year-old father-in-law, who received a hard sell about getting an accommodative intraocular lens implant when his cataract is removed, so that he will not need glasses. This is in spite of the fact that he has worn glasses without complaint most of his life, and an extra $2,800 per eye will have to be paid out of his pocket, since this new procedure is not covered by Medicare. All these things help emphasize the need for a book like mine, which is written from a patients' viewpoint of being able to understand enough about their eyes so as not to be confused or undeservedly swayed by such statements.

When talking to friends, other doctors, and patients, I have become progressively impressed that people do not understand simple basic facts about their eyes. This extends from the need for glasses, health of the eye, eye diseases, and alternatives available for seeing better. Many people are unnecessarily concerned about their eyes, and others are not even concerned enough to get their eyes examined to see if they need glasses or have eye disease. Parents need to know how to provide good eye care for their children, and themselves, when they inevitably are candidates for visual help, usually glasses. The news and advertisements currently are full of "new discoveries" and techniques to "improve vision," usually by "laser." It will be helpful to understand how the eye works so as to not be misled by claims to make the eyes better. Age-related eye problems need understanding. I hope to provide a book that is something people will want to read, cover to cover, and not the typical reference book that is full of things difficult to understand.

My plan is to give some basic information in a way so that people can not only educate themselves, but are also able to appreciate the nature of their eye problems, or potential eye problems. I want to attract attention of those who have no eye problems, but want to be alert for early treatment or avoidance of problems. For those who have eye abnormality, I hope to explain details of eye care so that a person is less mystified, and also help inform those whose duty it is to care for those handicapped by eye disorder with eye problems. If I can also provide a reference book that can be used to evaluate and understand current events in eye care, it should be easier for people to understand new developments when they are reported. In presenting the facts as they are, I also discuss areas of controversy, not only in the management of eye problems, but among the caregivers themselves. Hopefully, this will stimulate discussion, understanding, and the intent to improve on the means of providing eye care.

Ultimately, I hope to present an encouraging picture about the present status of excellence in eye care and excitement about future potential. Much of what I have to say is based on what I have learned as an ophthalmologist over a period of forty-five years. Some of what I have to say is based on my personal opinions, and not necessarily shared by all eye doctors. In general, however, my principles of treatment can be considered traditional and in line with mainstream medicine. This is not a textbook, and if further information is desired, more detailed information is available from your eye doctor, the library, or the Internet. Most of the information included in this book is based on how I would explain things to my patients, off the top of my head (spontaneous), and straight from the shoulder (factual).

PART I

THE BASICS

1

Anatomy: Eye Structure and Function

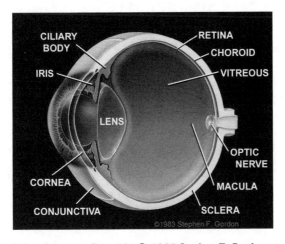

Parts of the eye. Copyright © 1983 Stephen F. Gordon.

To begin to understand the eye, one might make a simple anatomical comparison to a camera and its parts. The eye of course is relatively round and filled with fluids. It grows along with the rest of the body and reaches full size about the same time as the rest of the body becomes fully developed. If of average size, like most, the eye is "emmetropic," and is like a camera already in focus for distance, or "infinity" in math terms. An eye longer than average would be "nearsighted," or "myopic," and is in focus at a closer distance. The measurements in optical terms are in "diopters" and in the metric system. For example, a 3 diopter nearsighted eye is in focus at 1/3 meter, its far point.

Focusing, or accommodation, in the eye is an automatic feature, as in a point-and-shoot camera, which can automatically adjust its focus as required. At 1/3 meter, an emmetropic eye, like a camera already in focus for distance, would have to change its focus automatically, by 3 diopters. The farsighted eye is smaller than average, and if 3 diopters "hyperopic," it must focus automatically 3 diopters to see for distance, and another 3 diopters to see an object at 1/3 meter. Since the youthful eye can change its focus up to 10 diopters, only a nearsighted person may be aware of vision problems at a young age, as trouble seeing at a distance, like the "chalk board" in school. The eye cannot "unfocus" in a way to improve distance vision for the nearsighted. If a person is 3 diopters nearsighted, 1/3 meter is the far point, and anything closer than 1/3 meter requires focusing, but anything further away is progressively blurred.

By the way, the size of the eye is not so obvious to others. We estimate this size by how wide the eyelids are open. So persons with droopy lids look as if they have small eyes, and conversely those whose eyes are wide open (as in wide-eyed youth) appear to have large eyes. The "bug-eyed" appearance of someone with a hyperactive thyroid gland is due to the eyelids being unusually wide open, or due to upper lid retraction, and the eye may also become pushed forward, resulting in a condition called exophthalmos. Coincidentally, the glasses worn to correct vision by the nearsighted person with anatomically larger eyes make the eyes appear smaller (minified). And conversely, the glasses worn to correct vision by the farsighted person with smaller eyes make the eyes appear larger (magnified). You can tell if persons are nearsighted or farsighted when they have their glasses on by looking at their profile through the glasses they are wearing. The side of the face lateral to the eye appears indented, or minified, when a nearsighted person wearing fairly strong glasses is viewed from the front, and the lens of the glasses is thicker on the edge. The farsighted person's profile is more magnified, or bowed outward, when viewed from the front, and the lens is thicker in the center than at the edge.

How does the eye change its focus? It is obviously something going on internally, since the eye is relatively rigid and cannot change its size to account for needs of focusing. The very front of the eye is the cornea. Behind the cornea is the pupil forming iris tissue, the colored part of the eye as seen from the front. Behind the pupil is the lens of the eye, which brings things into focus, like the lens of a camera. The lens can change shape to become more powerful as focusing is required, especially when we are young. The rigidity of the lens increases with age, resulting eventually in focusing problems, and, in the extreme, causes cataract. Loss of focusing ability as we age is, in theory, a source of controversy. However, most agree that it is *not* due to the weakening of our "focusing muscles." The Helmholz theory is the most accepted, and this suggests that focusing takes place by means of the zonules, which are guy wires holding the lens in place and connected around the circumference of the eye to the ciliary body, a muscular tissue located behind the pupil. When the focusing muscles of the ciliary body work, they actually make the zonular connecting wires relax, and this allows the lens to round up and become more magnifying by becoming thicker in the center. When the lens becomes more rigid, it cannot round up as well with the ciliary muscle effort. When the ciliary muscles relax, the zonules become tighter and return the lens to the normal shape at rest. The nearsighted eye remains nearsighted. The lens of the eye cannot become thinner than usual; it cannot "unfocus."

The cornea is the clear, rounded front part of the eye. If we think of the eye as a ball, such as a tennis ball, then the cornea is like a clear blister on the front surface. Since it is transparent, it cannot be seen with the naked eye, unless a person is viewed from the side. Then the clear bulge can be seen in profile. This is an unusual tissue, since it has no blood vessels. The cornea externally receives nutrition from tears and the aqueous fluid bathing its internal surface. Nevertheless, when healthy, it transmits light as clearly as glass. If diseased or scarred, it may be invaded by blood vessels and then become opaque like the "white" of the eye, the sclera. Scars or opacities of the cornea may make vision similar to looking through a dirty window. Although the cornea could be compared to the lens cover in a camera, the human cornea has a much greater function. Being rounded in curvature, it actually plays an important role in focusing light to the back of the eye—the retina—an average of 24 millimeters away. However, unlike the lens of the eye, the cornea cannot change shape to focus the eye. Nevertheless, the curvature of the cornea can be surgically changed, and that is the basis of most "refractive surgery." The cornea is also the only part of the eye that can be transplanted, as in a corneal transplant surgery performed for corneal injury or disease.

If the cornea is out of round, more football shaped than basketball spherically shaped, we speak of astigmatism. Since most of us are not perfect, most of us have some astigmatism. This is no big deal in most cases, not initially effecting the need for glasses unless accompanied by significant nearsightedness or farsightedness. However, a higher degree of astigmatism can be an important factor in correcting vision to an acceptable degree. We speak of farsighted, nearsighted, and mixed astigmatism, on the basis of its effect in addition to the basic "refractive error." Although, technically, astigmatism makes vision imperfect at any distance, minor degrees of astigmatism may not be much of a factor in needing glasses, until one develops presbyopia, the age-related need for reading glasses. You can estimate the degree of astigmatism in persons by holding their glasses in front of a vertical or horizontal line and rotating the lens. If the line stays straight, then there is little or no astigmatism correction, but if the line bends it is due astigmatism correction in the glasses.

When light strikes the cornea, the most forward outward part of the eye, it is then transmitted through the "pupil." Actually, the pupil is just a black-looking, round space formed by the colored part of the eye, the iris. The pupil functions like an aperture, in a camera, becoming larger in reduced light to let more light in, and smaller in bright light so as to protect the delicate interior of the eye from "overexposure." The pupil has no focusing effect, it just controls how much light getting to the back of the eye. The size of the pupil may vary among individuals, and still be normal.

Normally, pupils are of equal size, with some exceptions. Difference in size may be congenital, but if acquired, it should be reported as something of possible significance neurologically. Normally, the pupil should be able to promptly change size—for example, to become smaller when exposed to bright light. When young, our pupils are larger on average, but become smaller with age. Their size may be affected by medications, such as pilocarpine, used for treating glaucoma sometimes, and which makes the pupil small, or "miotic." Sometimes people with small (miotic) pupils have better vision than expected without glasses, for both near and distant objects, because of the "pinhole effect." However, larger pupils can be a sign of drug use, and something police officers look for—for example, at a traffic stop.

As mentioned, the pupil is formed by the iris, or the "colored part" of the eye. In regulating the pupil size, or aperture, the iris also serves as a "blackout drape" to protect the interior of the eye from overexposure to light. The muscles in the iris control the pupil size. Viewed through a microscope, called a slit lamp, the front of the iris appears diaphanous and irregular on the surface. Contrary to popular opinion, there are no such things as green, hazel, or blue eyes. Composed of two layers, the iris has a dense, black-pigmented "blackout drape" on its posterior; this layer is the same in all races. It is the front layer that gives the impression of various eye colors. The front layer is irregular on the surface and may vary from purely white to shades of brown. White superficially superimposed onto black gives the appearance of blue eyes: the whiter the front layer, the bluer the eye appears. Various shades of brown are determined by how much brown pigment is sprinkled on the front surface of the iris. A light dusting of brown pigment can give a yellowish appearance, and this yellow plus blue yields the green appearance.

The idea that the color of the eye changes depending on what you wear in clothing is therefore not true. Instead, the eye color changes depending on the size of the pupil. In bright light, the pupil is small, and what pigment is on the front surface is rather scattered and spread out, making the eye color lighter, looking like, but never quite really, "green" or "hazel." When larger, the pupil size causes the pigment to be compressed together, making the eye color darker. Of course, the dense pigment of the front surface results in dark brown eyes. Albinos, who lack pigment in all tissues, of course have blue eyes, and the albinism may be limited to the eyes, as in ocular albinism. Myths about the importance of eye color shades have led to various claims, including a pseudoscience called "iridology," which is something similar to reading one's palms.

The lens of the eye is a biconvex (thick in the middle and tapered at the edges) protein-layered gel that is optically clear in youth. It becomes more rigid in consistency and less clear with age. This rigidity apparently results in focusing problems of an age-related nature, called presbyopia, and in advanced degree, cataract formation. A cataract is a clouding of the normal lens that obstructs the amount of light passing on to be focused on the retina (comparable to the film in a camera), lining the back of the eye. The opacity of the lens may be nuclear (central), cortical (peripheral), or posterior subcapsular (such as opacity painted on the back of the lens). Variations of process occur, but it can be said that we all develop cataracts, if we live long enough. Some would have to be well over 100 before they might need cataract surgery. Of course, many die before having notable problems from cataracts. However, there is also no such thing as being too old for cataract surgery, if needed. And since the age expectancy of our population is increasing, cataract surgery is, and should continue to be, the most common surgery performed in the United States. But fear not: cataract surgery will be found to be not so bad; in fact it is much easier to tolerate than most surgical procedures. When performed once truly needed, it can be most rewarding to both patient and ophthalmologist. Cataract surgery will be discussed in more detail later.

Behind the lens is a relatively large cavity, the core of the eye, filled with the vitreous fluid. This is a thick, clear gel made up mainly of water. Its function, other than filling up space and providing nutrition perhaps, is largely unknown after its role in developing the congenital eye structure. Since clear, it optically transmits light via the pupil and lens onto the retina. It can be replaced with a waterlike fluid, when necessary in surgery, such as when removing a hemorrhage from the vitreous. Opacities may form in this fluid, and are called floaters, since they move around in the thick gel.

The retina is a thin layer of nerve tissue lining the inside of the back two-thirds of the eye, like wallpaper. It is comparable to the film in a camera, with exceptions. Unlike camera film, the retina has varying sensitivity. It is made up of cells called rods and cones, which are specialized in function. The small area in the center of the back of the eye, where light is focused, is called the macula. It occupies the back apex of the eye, where light is brought into focus. It is composed of 100 percent cones, which specialize in reading vision, color, and form vision. The percentage of cones gradually diminishes in areas of the retina more peripheral from the macula, mixing with cells called rods, until, in the peripheral retina, there are mainly rods. The rod cells are important for night vision, motion sensation, and peripheral vision. Retinal diseases involving the macula and the peripheral retina will be discussed later in this book.

The optic nerve, the second cranial nerve, enters the back of the eye, toward the nose from the macula, as a direct extension of the brain. Nerve fibers from the retina bunch up and travel along the optic nerve, giving visual impulses to the brain. The brain is "so smart" that it reverses upside-down images resulting from the cameralike eye into right-side-up images. The left side of the brain sees things to the right, and the right side of the brain sees everything to the left. Glaucoma affects the optic nerve, as do other diseases such as optic neuritis. Like brain tissue, it may not recover from a prolonged lack of oxygen, which can occur slowly in diseases such as diabetes, or from a sudden blockage in the circulation of the central retinal artery or vein.

2

EYE DEVELOPMENT AND CONGENITAL EYE PROBLEMS

We are not born with 20/20 vision. Hearing ability probably precedes vision to account for the apparent parental recognition from the baby bed. By age three months, infants can fixate on and follow a penlight or follow the parents around the room with their eyes. Vision levels possible because of the macular portion of the retina—that is, to be able see colors and small objects as little as newsprint—usually take six months to develop. Unfortunately, there are situations that may delay or prevent normal vision development, such as being cross-eyed, having congenital cataracts, congenital glaucoma, nystagmus (dancing eyes), severe myopia (nearsightedness), or other birth anomaly.

As mentioned, beginning in childhood, there are imperfections in the un-aided visual performance of the eyes. Most eyes are farsighted in childhood, because they are not fully grown and therefore smaller than the average reached by an adult. Compensating for this, the young have tremendous powers of accommodation, so focusing is not a problem at any distance for most children. Some are born nearsighted, (congenital myopia), and can be expected to become more nearsighted with growth. Although nearsightedness (myopia) is usually considered just a variation of normal vision, those who are congenitally myopic may be so to such a severe degree as to have degenerative problems later. Since eyes change with growth, the originally farsighted children tend to become less farsighted, with most eventually reaching relative emmetropia, in being able to focus for distance without effort. Some change enough to become myopic or nearsighted, and this condition can be expected to be progressive throughout growth, and also eventually stabilizing. The younger the onset of nearsightedness, the more rapid progress.

All children should be screened visually before kindergarten. Those whose parents have special eye problems, such as being cross-eyed or having a "lazy eye," should be screened by age three. Also be warned that a hereditary eye problem may skip a generation, so that if any grandparents have a history of a lazy eye, the rule still applies for early screening. A preschool child who is a little nearsighted, may not need glasses, but can be expected to become more nearsighted with growth. So in a year or so, the child may need glasses, and this is good to know so as to avoid problems in school. Parents who are also nearsighted may not be so surprised, having gone through the same stages during school-age development. Some parents, especially those who did not need glasses in school, are surprised at, and sometimes interested in, anything that can prevent the usual myopic development. Not realizing that there are no exercises to make the eye smaller, such parents are easily influenced by false claims about eye exercises or other ideas that may stop the progression of myopia. Of course, refractive surgery is not usually practical for the young. As researched at the Mayo Clinic, the most successful treatment to limit the development of myopia that I know about, is the use of atropine. Atropine paralyzes focusing and has to be used for years during growth. During this time the child must wear bifocals so as to be able to read. In general, this has not been a very popular treatment. A new experimental medicine, called pirenzepine, has been tried, but it has not yet been proven to be effective for limiting myopic development.

Part of the misunderstanding about nearsightedness is the idea that the myopic or nearsighted eye is "weak." This, of course, is not true. Eyes are not "weak" or "strong." They are of average size, larger, or smaller. And since when has being bigger than average meant weakness? The reason for this is largely genetic, and not environmental. People do not become nearsighted from reading too much, reading in poor light, or wearing their glasses too much.

The average child has no problem accepting glasses, though their parents may be a source of resistance. This acceptance is especially true if the child is young, when they are quite adaptable. The blurred distance vision of children may rather sneak up on them. Their first clue may be problems seeing things at the "board" that other classmates can see. Not knowing what is "normal," the nearsighted child is often amazed to see leaves on trees, and other things they did not know they were missing, when they get their first glasses. Acceptance of glasses may be not so good, if the first experience is later, like in junior high or high school. A negative attitude may occur due to "presumed" peer reaction, and the choice of contact lenses may be requested by the student, instead of glasses. However, the first glasses are usually not too strong, and contact lenses are for those who need stronger, full-time glasses, in general. Another factor is that an immature attitude toward glasses may also make contact lenses an expensive alternative, if they are not worn. My approach is to always to insist on glasses as the first alternative. Then, if the children demonstrates that they really like seeing as well as they do with glasses, but would rather not wear glasses, they may switch to contact lenses, usually at the next annual exam. There is no age limit, but age thirteen or so is a practical time to begin contact lenses. Girls are better than boys, because of dexterity, attitude, and general motivation. However, we also have several successful patients younger than thirteen, usually girls. In general, there seems to be a wide range of maturity in children, relative to contact lens wear.

CONGENITAL EYE PROBLEMS

Babies do not initially see well. They do not see well enough to fixate and follow, such as to a penlight, until age three months. They cannot see color well or "read" until age six months, when their maculas develop. From that point the baby's vision is relatively good, unless complicated by congenital abnormality. These abnormalities may include cataracts, glaucoma, nystagmus, degenerative myopia, strabismus, and amblyopia.

Congenital cataracts are fortunately rare. If they are mild, of course, no surgery is needed, and there are reasons to postpone surgery as long as possible. Also, to be considered, however, is the fact that the visual result may be diminished, if the eye has never had a chance to see normally. Dense cataracts at birth create special problems. If the cataract only involves one eye, or at least is worse in one eye, then there is at least good prognosis for vision with the other eye, but the chances of the eye with cataract seeing well are quite poor, even after cataract surgery. Cataract surgery in children has always been more difficult in ways, but complicating the good result is the state of aphakia (no lens present). Thus extreme anisometropia (one eye being different from the other) resulted, meaning that the eye operated on is now quite farsighted (aphakik) and can not change focus. Under these circumstances, amblyopia (poor vision development) is very likely, even with treatment, including glasses, contact lenses, or patching. Although originally children were not considered candidates for intraocular lens implant with cataract surgery, the long-term results are now good enough to not contraindicate intraocular lens implants for the treatment of congenital cataracts. Potentially, by reducing anisometropia (difference between eyes), there is a better chance of decreasing amblyopia by utilizing intraocular implants, but the problem is still difficult to overcome. For example, does the brain know the difference between input from a pseudophakik eye and that from a "normal" eye?

Myopia can be present at birth, and when of high degree, it can be progressive and "degenerative" and complicated by macular damage. You can think of the problem as an eye so big, that "stretch marks" occur, and these can affect the central or macular vision. Retinal detachments are also more likely because of the stretching effect on the retina. These patients may not only need strong glasses, but may not be capable of normal vision, even with contact lenses or intraocular surgery. Fortunately, this degree of problem is unusual. It is interesting to understand that the complications of an extra large eye, even if visually improved by refractive surgery, still leave the eye structurally more susceptible to long-term complications such as retinal detachment, because of the stretching effect on the retina.

Congenital glaucoma, though rare, is usually far advanced before discovery. The first sign, unfortunately, may be enlargement of the infant's eye. Since the wall of the eye is relatively elastic during infancy, the eye may literally stretch as result of increased intraocular pressure. As expected, by this time it is usually too late to preserve vision, since the delicate optic nerve will already have been severely damaged.

Nystagmus, jerky movements of the eyes that prevent good vision, is one of the more common neurological problems present at birth. There are different types of nystagmus, varying from latent (sometimes), to constant, or even voluntary. Constant nystagmus is usually associated with subnormal vision. The eyes usually have horizontal, jerky movements, but nystagmus may be vertical or torsional (rotary). Some people can voluntarily move their eyes in a nystagmic fashion, and though they may be a source of entertainment at parties, they are not usually visually handicapped. Latent nystagmus means that ordinarily there is no nystagmus, but circumstances may bring it out—the most usual being when one eye is covered, such as in the course of an eye examination. For these people, we need to use ways of examining the eyes without covering one eye. A head turn may develop, if this allows the child to use the eyes together in this position of least nystagmus, and best vision. The degree of nystagmus can vary, as well as the limitation of vision. The vision may be good enough to get a child through primary, and often secondary, school in regular classes. Low-vision programs are available in many schools. In grade school, the print in books is often large enough to allow a child with subnormal vision to manage. There may be other eye problems, such as optic nerve disease, but the child is otherwise usually normal neurologically.

Strabismus is the most common of the congenital problems, but is not always evident from birth. The worst complication is amblyopia, (poor vision development), or lazy eye, which is usually associated with esotropia, the crossing or inward turning of one eye. Exotropia, or outward-turning of one eye, in early childhood may have more serious neurological significance, since the straying of a blind eye is expected to be inward (crossed) in childhood. I recall suggesting to parents of an infant with exotropia that a neurologic problem may be present, and unfortunately I was correct, he had a brain tumor. Treatment will be discussed with various types of strabismus. in chapter seven.

Anisometropia is a condition in which one eye is different from the other, for example, one eye may be farsighted, and the other may have astigmatism or nearsightedness. Next to being cross-eyed, this is the second-most common cause of amblyopia (lazy eye). In a way, these anisometropic children are worse off than being cross-eyed, because their parents are usually unaware of any eye problem until initial vision screening, usually after the child has started school. By this time, treatment is often too late. Of prime import is a family history of lazy eye among siblings, parents, grandparents, aunts, and uncles. Any such history should alert parents to having their child examined at least by age three. After that, the result of treatment may be poor, whereas early treatment of amblyopia can result in normal vision. If initiated early, patching, glasses, or eye drops may help develop vision. Apparently, the natural thing for the eyes to do is to pick the eye that sees best without glasses and to preferentially focus with this eye for best vision. The eyes apparently focus equally, so that if one eye sees well with minimal focusing, this eye is in focus and the other may be left blurred. Therefore, vision in the blurred eye does not develop fully. Contrary to popular myths, the "weak eye" does not become "stronger" should something happen to the good eye.

Retinopathy of prematurity (ROP) is a complication for extremely small, premature babies, such as those less than two pounds at birth, but was more common in years past, when unregulated amounts of oxygen were given to incubator babies. The severity can vary, but treatment is usually necessary to preserve a degree of useful vision.

3

Vision Testing and Problem Treatment

Vision testing can begin with vision screening. Such vision screening can be performed by nonprofessional personnel, for preschool or regular school purposes, as long as it is understood that such screening does not replace a professional eye examination. A preschool child can learn to do the "illiterate E game," usually after reaching age three. This test involves an eye chart composed entirely of the letter E, turned in different directions, and, like a regular "Snellen" eye chart, arranged in rows of smaller and increasing difficulty. Someone who can't read English, or a small child, can learn to point which way the "fingers" point on the letter E. A difference in performance between eyes would suggest the need for a professional exam to rule out need for glasses or amblyopia. Screening tests utilizing the usual Snellen charts can also be performed later once of school age, and are likely to be more accurate in discovery of vision problem. Failure, of course, would suggest the need for a professional exam, even though the screening tests may still be inaccurate. Passing the vision screen is reassuring and suggests no significant distance vision problem or serious astigmatism. However, these tests cannot detect reading problems, the history of which suggests the need for seeing an eye doctor. Certainly, a family history of eye problems, including the need for glasses, is helpful in determining the need for a professional exam.

Modern screening tests now include photoscreening and photorefractors, new technologies that may work well with small children, but whose current availability may make them impractical for large-scale screening of children. Generally, I favor school eye-screening exams, and wish that they be more universally available. As the National Institute of Health (NIH) recently inferred, trained lay personnel can quite effectively perform preschool screening exams. However, there is some controversy as regards the need for legislated professional eye exams, which are proposed by some. Unfortunately, those who propose these exams are often likely to overdiagnose and overprescribe glasses, as studies show. One study showed that 34 percent of professionally screened children, as would be the case via forced legislation, were given glasses, whereas only 3 percent of this same test group had glasses recommended by a pediatric ophthalmologist. However, I agree that overreferral for eye exams—for example, of children who are not performing the screening test to their capability—is preferable to overlooking children who need attention.

Reading disabilities, of at least some degree, are very common among young schoolchildren. This creates concern among parents and teachers, but problematically, these conditions are frequently overemphasized and overdiagnosed. It is too easy to blame lack of performance on some special problem that requires special treatment. For example, the term "dyslexia" is greatly overused, whereas it is really a quite rare condition whereby reading may persist as a problem throughout life. Most reading and learning disabilities respond to patience and special attention and do not require the type attention needed for true dyslexia. In other words, extra schooling in reading skill will usually help most children who are initially slow to learn, and many children are wrongly labeled as requiring specialist attention. Dyslexia and attention deficit disorder (ADD) are both terms that are often overused, but it is understandable how parents and teachers are quick to reach for any help available for a child. Unfortunately, some weird forms of treatment have surfaced, such as eye exercises, creeping and crawling methods, and red-tinted glasses. Another theory has suggested that a child with cross-dominance, for example a child who fixates with the left eye, though right-handed, may have resultant reading problems. However, studies of those without reading problems would show the same incidence of cross-dominance. Certainly the patching in attempt to change the dominance is fruitless. Since there is a very good prognosis for improvement of all reading disorders with any special attention to the problem, apparent improvement is often falsely taken as a sign that such things as eye exercises deserve credit for the improvement. As for glasses, it is probably best to error on the side of treatment in "borderline" indications rather than ignore any possible help for the child with a reading disorder. But, in most cases, it is an oversimplification, and usually a false diagnosis, to blame reading and learning disorders as due to eye abnormality.

What about sports, and indication for glasses or other treatment in athletics? Young people involved in athletics need some guidance. Visual needs vary per sport. For example, a boy who is 1 diopter nearsighted may perform OK without glasses in soccer, football, and basketball. But in baseball, where he has to see to hit the fast-moving smaller ball, or in tennis, especially at night, where he has to play under lights, the glasses may well be appreciated. The more nearsighted child may need glasses for all sports. The farsighted child or those with moderate astigmatism may perform well without glasses in most sports. Ask your eye doctor if it is really necessary for this child to wear the glasses in sports? Another problem, of course, is that the glasses may get in the way, fall off, or get broken. Special sports glasses frames are helpful, and when the child becomes old enough, contact lenses may be substituted. Because of rumors of super vision in athletes, such as Ted Williams, there may be offers of special exercises or glasses to give super vision. Actually, many people are able to see better than 20/20 with or without glasses, and this capability cannot be taught or improved upon once eye maturity is reached. I believe that certain athletes have the gift of super concentration, along with good eye–hand coordination, and this results in their apparent visual excellence. I doubt that this coordination can be taught, but I am sure concentration can be improved with experience.

Among the latest practices, encouraged by professional baseball players, is the wearing of colored contact lenses (red) and utilizing a technique of watching tennis balls with numbers painted on them. By concentrating on seeing the numbers, someone able to hit the ball could be expected to perform better in baseball or tennis. Rather than claim super vision, I think this is an example of learning to increase concentration.

The detection of amblyopia, or lazy eye, is one of the main reasons for vision screening in preschool children. The amblyopic eye is structurally normal, but does not see well even with glasses. People often mistakenly refer to a lazy eye as one that does not appear straight and seems to wander. The eye's turning inward toward the nose is esotropia (cross-eyed) and turning outward is exotropia (walleyed). The most common cause of amblyopia is being cross-eyed, and if one eye is noted to be always the one crossed, then this one does not see well. The second-most common cause of amblyopia is anisometropia, in which one eye that "needs glasses" is significantly different from the better eye. In a way, the cross-eyed child is more fortunate in the treatment of amblyopia, because the parents can see suggestive evidence that the child's eyes are not normal. In anisometropia, too often the problem is not discovered until the child is in school and too old to be treated successfully. Amblyopia can be mild, or so bad as to be legally blind, with no hope of ever seeing better with the "bad eye." The "site" of amblyopia is in the brain, not the eye, and this has been experimentally proved in animals to be incomplete development of the lateral geniculate body. The eye looks perfectly normal anatomically, even with careful examination. Apparently, in order to avoid double vision, the brain suppresses, or turns off, the central portion of vision. This means that, contrary to the closing of one eye, the peripheral vision is retained, so that people with amblyopia can have enough side vision to function well while driving a car and in most sports, retaining a form of binocular vision. But if something ever happened to their good eye, the second-best eye would never improve for reading and for things that require good vision. In early childhood, the brain is relatively flexible and able to ignore the central vision in one eye so as to avoid confusion, as might be caused by double vision. The eye most perfect in focus is usually chosen because it is the easiest to use. The eyes do not apparently focus separately, so if 2 diopters of focusing is required in one eye, and 5 diopters in the other eye, the lesser amount of focusing is chosen, which leaves the more farsighted eye out of focus due to anisometropia. It is interesting that if both eyes need glasses rather badly, vision development seems to take place equally well, and vision may be relatively normal once glasses are prescribed, even when one is older. However, in some cases, if a significant uncorrected refractive error is present until adult life, both eyes may not see perfectly well, even with corrective glasses.

The treatment of amblyopia amounts to forcing the child to use the nonpreferred eye. This amounts to covering the "good eye," usually by an adhesive eye patch. The sooner the treatment is begun, the better the expected result. Many newborns have relatively wandering and nonfocusing eyes. Babies do not usually fixate well, such as to a light or object, until about three months old, and vision is quite immature until six months old. So if the baby's eyes are always crossed or not straight, a professional eye exam is indicated. However, if the eyes only sometimes don't look straight, it is OK to wait. But if the baby is six months old, and a parent still thinks the eyes look crossed, or not straight, even if just sometimes, then it is not too soon to get the baby examined. At such an early age, patching may not take long to help. And we don't have to wait until the child knows the alphabet to confirm success. The ability to fixate and hold fixation with each eye, on a doctor's penlight for example, helps demonstrate that better vision has developed.

Patching may seem cruel to some parents, and they may not be good about enforcing the rule of patching all the waking hours. Some children are more difficult to deal with than others. Problems in patching should be discussed with the eye doctor so the doctor is not so surprised when it doesn't seem to be working. Medical patching may be done using atropine eye drops to dilate the good eye so that its temporary lack of focusing ability makes it seem undesirable to use compared with the amblyopic eye, which can still focus normally. This has to be carefully supervised by the eye doctor, but does not require so much cooperation. Recent studies have shown that it may only be necessary to use atropine drops on weekends, on children of up to age seven. However, most patching is relatively unsuccessful by the time the child is in kindergarten, and it is debatable whether this is due to the fact that it is too late (the brain's being is too well developed), or due to a combination of lack of enthusiasm of the child, parents, and teachers. Performance in school is held as supreme in goal, and failure of a child to meet expectations in school may be blamed on the patching.

What is a good result of the treatment of amblyopia? Well, any improvement helps assure less handicap should something happen to the better eye. Sustained visual development in childhood means that this vision will always be available in the nonpreferred eye, no matter which way the eye points, like money in the bank. The contrary—that the eye may develop vision later if needed—is, unfortunately, not true. The best the eye will ever see is what it could see with corrective glasses in early school age. Another reason to try to get normal vision is that in the case of the cross-eyed child who needs surgery to straighten the eyes, the only hope of attaining normal binocular vision is to have equally good vision in both eyes. If one eye is still the second-best eye, then even though the eyes are straightened, they will not be used well binocularly. Also, the permanence of the surgical result is affected, since binocularity helps hold the eyes together as a team. Lack of binocularity may result in eventual relative failure of the surgery, sometimes resulting in the need for further surgery for cosmetic reasons.

Binocular vision apparently develops normally between age five and nine and can be described as stereoptic vision. In other words, the depth perception available normally to those with normal stereopsis would mean that lack of this would make the 3-D glasses unhelpful for 3-D movies. Also, binoculars would not be as useful. However, there are degrees of binocular vision, so that even those with amblyopia, who "suppress" vision in one eye to avoid double vision, do retain peripheral vision, to attain a kind of gross binocularity. This, of course, makes a big difference in sports and car driving. There are also monocular clues for judging distance, such as converging parallel lines suggesting distance that artists use in paintings.

What if the treatment of amblyopia is unsuccessful, too late, or too little? Well, it is not the end of the world. Certainly, it is important to try our best to achieve the best vision possible. However, if we all tried our best, that is as good as we can do. Most importantly, as long as one eye is normal in vision development, there is not expected to be any significant handicap in school or adult performances. The good eye will not wear out, and it is under no great strain to "do the work of two eyes." Other than perhaps major leaguer baseball, I can't think of any sport where lack of 100 percent depth perception has been a significant handicap. I have personally examined a Hall of Fame pro basketball player, and a professional hockey league goalie, both of whom were only using one eye. About the only job restriction is of becoming an astronaut, because in "outer space" the lack of depth perception is more of a problem due to lack of monocular clues. And for sure, children with amblyopia are not to be considered handicapped, in any way. Reading disorders are not any more common with amblyopia. We expect normal school and athletic performances; no excuses. We are mainly concerned with the activities that involve increased danger of eye injury, such as in certain sports. One can get a driver's license, even if the "bad eye" sees no better than 20/200, with glasses. A problem could exist with the amblyopic person with anisometropia, if vision can be somewhat improved with glasses. But if a person is not used to wearing glasses because of marked difference between the eyes, your eye doctor can fill out a motor vehicle form to help, by pointing out that the glasses do not improve function, and may actually cause visual confusion.

Color blindness is not usually the chief complaint that leads to an eye exam, but is something easy to confirm by testing. Actually, such people are not "blind"; their vision is usually normal, but the problem is discrimination between shades of colors, usually in the red-green area, and not particularly handicapping. It is a sex-linked hereditary problem in most cases and affects about 5 percent of males in the United States of America. The trait is transmitted from their mothers, the "carrier" of the gene from her color-blind father. For example, the son of a color-blind man will not be color blind, or extend the tendency to his children. On the other hand, his sisters will extend the color-blind trait to all their sons. There are few limitations, as result of color blindness, except that mothers and wives must help pick out ties, and so forth. However, there are a few job limitations, as in electricians., for example. Female color blindness is rare; and when present, it may be accompanied with reduced vision.

USE OF DILATING EYE DROPS

Eye doctors use eye drops a lot. We use dilating eye drops to examine the retina, and other eye drops to treat most eye diseases. People have a natural aversion to eye drops, but can learn to use them as needed. In eye exams, pupil-dilating drops are used to get a better look of the eye's interior, as looking through a window rather than a keyhole.

It used to be true that one could tell the difference between an ophthalmologist, a medical eye doctor, and an optometrist, by the fact that the ophthalmologist always used dilating eye drops, during an eye exam but the optometrist did not. Now, optometrists, too, can use eye drops during the exam. Because they did not go to medical school, optometrists were restricted, and could not use or prescribe medication. Recent state laws have allowed use of medications, varying by state, but use of diagnostic medication such as dilating eyedrops are universally approved.

In children, especially young children, dilating the pupils is especially important in measuring the eyes' need for glasses objectively by a retinoscope. Because of cooperation limitations of children, objective measurement or estimation of need for glasses is extremely important, since they may have problems looking through instruments and maintaining attention. By using dilating drops, which relax the focusing of the eye, it is usually possible, if only briefly, to estimate objectively a young child's need for glasses. I have been routinely using such drops, especially for the initial exam, in all children under age eleven, unless prior exam has indicated that the child can do well without them subjectively. My dog, Bear, for example, was able to cooperate well enough: that while he sat still for me, I was able to tell with retinoscopy, that he did not "need glasses." However, he probably sat more still than most young children. Well, anyway, kids do not like eye drops, and it is helpful if the parents are prepared for them, and supportive. It is probably not a good idea to mention the eye drops before the exam, but it is helpful if the parents are firm and supportive when the eye drops are used. I usually say, "Nurse Nancy is going to put in some magic eye drops," and then leave. The kids are then mad at Nancy, and not me. When I return to finish the exam, I can reassure, "No more eye drops," and proceed.

Additional factors about children eye exams include relative frequent unreliability of their complaints. Normal child behavior has to be understood, before criticism in this discussion. Most children who complain of trouble seeing to read, or having headaches, usually do not have eye problems, or need glasses. On the contrary, those who do need help do not usually complain.

Those who need glasses often do not know what is normal vision, and problems can sneak up on them, especially on the nearsighted child. Trouble seeing things on the "board" can often be the first indication, when the child notes that other children their age can see the things on the "board" easily. Some of these nearsighted children can be noted to "squint" to see better, but excessive blinking of the eyes, squinting, and certain facial expressions are often just transient mannerisms, and not necessarily a sign of eye disease or need for glasses. The important thing is to have the child examined, and not be surprised if glasses are not indicated. Sometimes, however, it is also important to listen to consistent complaint, in spite of "normal" findings. Once, stuck for an answer to a boy in his early teens, I noted that he was taking acutane for his acne, and looked up the medicine in my Physician's Desk Reference. Sure enough, the drug can cause visual problems and headaches, which he described. His father, who accompanied the boy for a second opinion, was quite reassured to know that his son was not malingering, since he trusted in his son so much. Later, he called and told me that the symptoms had disappeared when the medicine was discontinued, which made me quite happy, too.

EXAMINATION OF THE EYES

The first basic part of an eye examination is to check vision. If vision is abnormal or subnormal, then a reason must be found. If the reason is that glasses are needed to see better, then this is reassuring. If glasses cannot correct the vision, then we must search for another reason. However, the degree of abnormality is the variation between best-corrected vision and normal vision, not by how poorly a person sees subjectively without glasses. So this point cannot be overemphasized: the basic, initial part of an eye examination is to see how well the eye can see. Sometimes the eyes are so obviously inflamed or injured as to indicate that the vision will be worse than usual, but we need to get an idea of how bad the problem affects the eye, on the basis of how poor the vision has become. We can always check for glasses when the eye is healthier, but we can get an idea of vision potential on initial examination. Potential for better vision can be estimated by what is called a pin-hole test. A disc filled with small holes allows a person to peek through one of the holes, and an improvement on how far down they can see on the Snellen chart suggests either that they need glasses or their present glasses are not correct, or that potential for better vision is present in the face of a cataract. A red eye due to "pink eye" usually does not affect vision, whereas a red eye due to glaucoma or iritis may be associated with drop in vision. Most vision testing, however, is in the course of routine eye examination, whereby a person may or may not complain of visual problems.

The measurement of vision and need for glasses is both subjective and objective. There are ways to measure vision potential, objectively, or the need for glasses, objectively. The most common is the retinoscope, an instrument used by the examiner with the refractor instrument or trial lenses in place. This is especially helpful in children and in all initial exams. Modern instrumentation has resulted in automatic refractors, machines that can relatively accurately measure the refractive state of the eye, the need for glasses. Sometimes these new machines can seem to shorten eye examination, so that commercial enterprises, à la those at malls, can quickly "grind out" your need for glasses. In office practice, however, eye doctors have always known that there is actually an "art" to refracting, and determining what glasses a patient may require. The subjective part of the exam involves asking patients what they appreciate as helpful to see best and the experience in knowing what responses are reliable. So the objective means of measuring vision is helpful, but the subjective portion of the exam is defining in terms of determining the presciption for glasses, if needed.

Included in the subjective "art" of refraction is the ability to detect when a patient response is inaccurate or inconsistent, because of intent, misunderstanding, or incapacity. In children, this is important. By the way, if a child does not do as well as is capable, or acts as if something is wrong, even if not so, this is not as serious as such performance when an adult does so, and is basically forgivable in an eye exam. Often, children are influenced by peers. In cases where an objective exam suggests no need for glasses but the child seems to demonstrate subnormal vision, trickery often works. By using patience and some trickery, it is often possible to "improve" the vision to normal with window-glass type glasses, meaning with little or nothing in the refractor machine. This is called a "toothpaste" refraction; you have to "squeeze it out of them." Sometimes trickery fails, and because of a lack of objective sign of a problem, the child and parents are reassured that no treatment is necessary. However, I have learned to suggest follow-up exam in at least one year to confirm things are OK, especially because of one patient.

Years ago, while working in a large multispecialty clinic, I examined a boy who was about twelve years old. His mother reported that a well-known ophthalmologist in the community had examined the child one or two years previously and had concluded that the child was not admitting how well he could see. In other words, the doctor was suggesting a form of conversion hysteria in the face of a normal eye exam. Because the boy's pediatrician was also in my clinic, I could read on the chart a sequence of events. The boy was referred to a psychiatrist, who concluded that the boy had a bad relationship with his father. The father was drawn into therapy in order to teach him how better to relate to his son, and was led to believe that such an improvement may help the child eventually see better. Influenced by this information, I was initially impressed by the boy's withdrawn attitude and the fact he diverted his gaze while talking, so as to not look me in the eye. Objective examination suggested the boy did not even need glasses, and subjectively I could not get him to admit better than 20/200 vision. Then I looked inside his eyes, at his retina, and practically cried. The poor boy had signs of macular degeneration, Stargardt's disease, and was never going to see normally, no matter how good his relationship became with his father. This type of macular disease in children becomes symptomatic before signs are evident in the eye, so the prior ophthalmologist had not been guilty of missing this diagnosis. The boy, however, was distraught when informed that he was not going to see better. He preferred the idea that someday his vision would improve, that the problem was all mental, and temporary. Later, the family moved to Michigan and an expert on Stargardt's disease, Dr. Harold Falls I believe, confirmed my diagnosis. The most important lesson I learned, though, was that if I cannot be sure that a child's eyes are probably normal, then I should suggest annual exams until we can demonstrate that the child can truly see normally. And I have never seen another case of Stargardt's disease.

External examination, of course, is important in screening for eye disease. The eyes are checked for anomalies of the pupils, eyelids, eye alignment, signs of inflammation, or peripheral vision limitation. The intraocular pressure is checked to screen for glaucoma. Microscopic examination is performed using a slit lamp, a magnifying device that allows examination of the cornea, anterior chamber, and lens, of the eye, and the anterior or front third of the eye. Many diseases can only be diagnosed with a slit lamp, such as iritis, herpes simplex corneal infections, corneal abrasions, contact lens complications, corneal opacities and foreign bodies, tear duct anomalies, or irritating eyelashes. General doctors trying to treat these conditions, are usually handicapped by not having the use of a biomicroscope, the slit lamp. An attachment to this instrument can also be used for measuring intraocular pressures.

Internal examination involves looking through the pupil, lens, and vitreous cavity to the back of the eye, the retina. This process is, called fundoscopy. A direct, ophthalmoscope or sometimes an indirect ophthalmoscope, is used. A cataract can obstruct view of the retina, as can any opacity of cornea or the vitreous cavity. The optic nerve is examined for signs of anomaly, including suggestive signs of glaucoma. The blood vessels around the optic nerve are scanned for signs of narrowing, which are suggestive of hypertensive arteriosclerotic disease. Signs of arteriolar narrowing, along with a history of hypertension being treated, can confirm the need for treatment. However, if the issue is described as "borderline," then signs of arteriolar narrowing suggest that the diagnosis should actually confirm hypertension is present, enough to warrant treatment. Any hemorrhages or exudates (edema patches) are to be noted; and they can be due to diabetes, hypertension, or other vascular problems. Screening exams for diabetic retinopathy are recommended annually, with the idea that vision threatened by diabetic retinopathy may need laser treatment. There are many retinal diseases that can be diagnosed with a direct, or indirect, ophthalmoscope, including macular degeneration, retinal detachment, retinitis pigmentosa, and other retinal degenerations.

Dilating the pupil is useful to better see inside the eye, as mentioned. Patients tend to be more concerned about this than necessary and often try to talk the eye doctor out of this part of the exam. Actually, dilating the pupil makes internal examination more like looking through a window (large pupil) rather than a keyhole (small pupil). Some young patients with naturally large pupils, can be examined without dilating the pupils, but if your eye doctor suggests dilating them, your cooperation is suggested. As a result of dilating, vision can be blurred, but not so bad, especially if you have glasses that help. Reading is a bit blurred, for an hour or so, but if you are young, or if you have bifocals, there is not much of a problem. If the best-corrected vision is subnormal, then a search for cause is needed, and dilating the pupil is quite important in this search. And if you are nearsighted, you can remove your glasses to read. Sunglasses will be helpful for outdoors, and the eye doctor can provide temporary ones. People who have had cataract surgery sustain no visual blurring from dilation, since their focusing ability is not altered, though their customary feelings of sensitivity to light may make them reluctant to have their eyes dilated. In general, if your pupils have not been dilated for your eye examination, the exam may be incomplete.

Nonroutine additional exams may be recommended. For example, if glaucoma is suspected on the basis of family history, intraocular pressures, shallow anterior chambers, or cupping of the optic nerves, further tests may be indicated, such as a visual field or GDX (retinal nerve fiber testing). Suspected open-angle glaucoma requires such tests, since the diagnosis is often complicated, especially if the intraocular tension is not elevated. The visual field test is computerized, and helps detect early loss of vision due to glaucoma, before a patient would usually be aware of a problem. Early diagnosis, of course, is important in order to avoid further loss of vision. If narrow-angle potential glaucoma is suspected, then another test, called gonioscopy, may be performed. This test may help tell if prophylactic treatment for narrow-angle glaucoma is indicated. Photographs may be suggested for an evaluation of potential glaucoma or retinal diseases, such as macular degeneration. A retinal specialist often employs special photographic techniques, such as fluorescein angiography, a test that can be definitive in the diagnosis of diabetic retinopathy, macular degenerations, and other retinal diseases.

Medicare does not pay for routine eye examinations and for routine medical exams in general. The question is, what is routine? Medicare considers the checking of vision, "refraction," as routine and therefore denies payment for an eye exam, unless there is a medical diagnosis such as cataract. Then the refraction part, testing the vision, is "carved out," and the patient must pay for this portion of the exam. This seems especially unfair when it is recognized that testing the vision is so important in detecting the presence or severity of eye disease. For example, we measure cataracts by how much they reduce vision. It is also difficult to accept for many people, because they have become accustomed to vision coverage via union medical plans. Such plans are so common that once people reach Medicare age, they cannot understand why eye exams and glasses are not covered.

Guidelines for routine eye exams may be generalized. Probably all children should be examined prior to kindergarten. A family history of lazy eye would suggest even earlier examination, at age three or four. Once a child shows the need for glasses, annual exams are usually needed, because glasses take quite a beating, and growth may demonstrate change in the eyes and the need for prescription of glasses annually. It is hard to make rules for healthy young adults, especially if they do not need glasses, but by age forty, one should be examined at least every two years. Of course, if one uses glasses, then periodic exams seem obviously needed. The onset of diseases such as glaucoma, macular degeneration, and cataract increase in frequency significantly beyond age forty. People with diabetes need annual eye exams, so that early treatment can be initiated if needed. Contact lens wearers also need annual exams, and we follow cataract progress at least once a year. Glaucoma patients' need for exam, once they are under treatment, varies per patient and response to treatment, and with best control, it is usually no less than once yearly.

4

EYE GLASSES (SPECTACLES) AND CONTACT LENSES

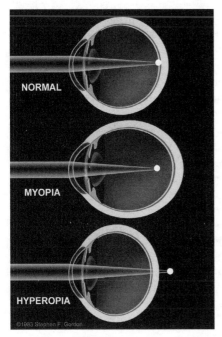

These illustrations show how light from far away (more than 20 feet) is focused onto the macula in the "normal" emmetropic eye. In the myopic eye, the light rays are bent by the cornea and lens in front of the macula, in an eye usually larger than average. A spectacle lens thicker on the edges would spread the light rays entering the eye enough to allow focus on the macula. The farsighted eye, being smaller than average, needs a spectacle lens thicker in the center to help bend light rays more so that they are in focus on the macula. Copyright © 1983 Stephen F. Gordon.

In general, as I will point out, we all need glasses eventually. Some are so shaken up by this fact that they seek other alternatives. I plan to discuss alternatives, but do not expect me to discourage the natural transition of need for glasses, spectacles if you wish, or may not wish.

As I mentioned, most of us are relatively emmetropic, meaning that we see quite well at all distances without glasses, at least while we are young adults and represent about 40 percent of the adult population. The nearsighted (myopic) usually begin to need glasses at an early age. The farsighted (hyperopic), child, unless more than 2 or 3 diopters farsighted, functions well in school and generally. However, they may demonstrate a problem reading earlier than emmetropic presbyopes, perhaps in the twenties or thirties. Presbyopia, the physiological loss of focusing vision, can be predicted. Between age forty and forty-five, the average emmetrope, meaning most of us, will notice the "arms too short" problem. This statement, of course, is due to the fact that holding things closer, as we used to do as children to see better, actually makes things worse, since the closer we hold things, the more is the demand for focusing. At about age forty-five, the maximum focusing ability is down to about 3.5 diopters. Therefore, reading at 1/4 meter (16 inches), which demands a 2.5-diopters accommodation, is more difficult. It is natural, then, to hold things farther away, which requires less focusing effort. Also, good light helps, which explains why people move over to the window to read. We refer to the need for "reading glasses," but actually we are talking about seeing any small object up close, as in sewing, or working with small screws or nails.

The need for help seeing at near is predictable and common to all, but some terms are confusing. Some say, "You get farsighted in your forties." Not true. We all become presbyopic, and this is added to one's original basic refractive status. Therefore, if you are basically nearsighted, you too become presbyopic, and when wearing your distance glasses, you eventually notice that you must hold things farther away to read, with your glasses on. Removing the glasses makes things seen better, depending on how nearsighted you are. The same is true for those wearing contact lenses: close work becomes difficult, and removing contact lenses is not so convenient for the nearsighted.

What is hard to understand for the emmetrope is the eventual need for glasses, when everything has seemed perfect. However, the most disappointed person is the farsighted one. Being "farsighted," a person may think that the more farsighted one is, the farther away one can see. Wrong. The more farsighted one is, the more one needs to focus, even for distance, and therefore when presbyopic loss of focusing develops, most of these people have also lost distance vision. And because they used to see so well for distance, they have trouble accepting the fact that they have developed primarily a reading problem, but now secondarily also a distance problem. They may note friends who needed glasses in school for nearsightedness, but who now can often still see well up close by taking their glasses off. However, the farsighted person may reach a point where glasses are needed full time, to see both near and distance objects, and this may not seem fair.

We can predict, within limits, when the presbyopia-driven need for glasses will occur. Drugstore, or over-the-counter, glasses are available, so that we can use the terms of spectacle power expectations. Of course, these glasses assume that both eyes are the same and that there is no significant need for astigmatism correction. However, most people do not fit this category. These glasses are, also made to be relatively "one size fits all," so that the distance between pupils is not such as to allow for variables, and the frame in general may not fit well. Between ages forty and forty-five, the weakest power of +1.00 is needed by the emmetrope or a person wearing contact lenses. Later, by age fifty, a +1.75 or +2.00 power will be needed. By age sixty or so, a +2.25 reading power, and the full power of +2.50, meaning the full power for seeing at 1/4 meter, is eventually needed.

An interesting point: if a person finds that he or she can see well for distance with drugstore reading glasses, then something is obviously wrong, right? Well, I have been in contact with two "professional" people recently, who use drugstore reading glasses for distance. The nurse uses +2.50, usually the strongest available for watching TV, and the chiropractor uses +1.75, for tennis. The nurse was told by the DMV that she needed to wear her +2.50 readers for driving and stated so on her license. Neither understood the implication of this phenomenon. Now, do you? It means that both are significantly farsighted. So, as a rule, if people notice that they can see well for distance with drugstore reading glasses, then they are farsighted enough to definitely need bifocals, or another alternative if they are intent on avoiding glasses. The worst complication of choosing the over-the-counter reading glasses is that a person's satisfaction may be interpreted to mean that the eye problem has been solved and further eye examination is not necessary. This ignores the fact that the same age-related problems revealing the need for help in reading also signifies the need for screening for eye diseases such as glaucoma, cataract, macular degeneration, and other such age-related potential problems.

Those who are interested in cosmetics would be likely interested in the no-line bifocal, the progressive add. Since there is no obvious line separating the distance from the reading portion of the lens, they look like single-vision glasses, therefore hiding the "stigma" of being old enough to need bifocals. However, if they have been using single-vision drugstore glasses, the progressives may be difficult to deal with because the reading area is relatively smaller. More than once, having presented the better choice of bifocals over single-vision reading glasses, I have been surprised by patients' response that they are already using bifocal sunglasses, which they also got at the drugstore. On this subject, it can be pointed out that one's regular bifocal or progressive lenses can have "transitions," the ability to darken outside and lighten up again back inside, a very good option for those wanting to simplify the number of pairs of glasses.

When informed of the eventual need for glasses, different and sometimes extreme patient reactions occur. One lady, when informed of the impending need for reading glasses, had a reaction similar to Andy of London, a comic-strip character. Andy stated that he was so sick and tired of reading that drinking is bad for your health that he was going to quit. When asked if he was then going to quit drinking, he said no, he was going to quit reading. My patient said the same. If she was going to need glasses, then she would just quit reading.

CONTACT LENSES

Contact lenses can be a substitute for glasses, but are usually worn by people who need relatively strong glasses. (I will use the terms "strong" and "weak," because people seem to understand these terms, though glasses and eyes are not strong or weak; rather, they are either more powerful or less powerful in focusing power.) The nearsighted are usually the the first candidates for contact lenses, even at a young age. The more nearsighted, the more motivated—girls more than boys for cosmetic reasons, but also boys for cosmetic and sports activities. The original contact lenses were "hard," lenses, rigid plastic lenses whose sphericity (roundness) also corrected astigmatism. The success rate was relatively unpredictable because they are rather uncomfortable, especially at first during the adjustment phase. Once successful with hard contact lenses, however, patients may be not satisfied with the relative lack of sharp vision, to which they are accustomed, if they try soft contact lenses. Nevertheless, soft contact lenses have taken over the majority of the contact lens market, because of initial and continued comfort, satisfactorily good vision, easy replacement, and relative safety.

Soft lenses feel better from the start, are safer healthwise, can be disposable, are usually worn all day long, but can be part-time. Extended wear is possible, but not encouraged without supervision (leave in place day and night for two to four weeks). Part-time wear is useful for those who wish to wear contact lenses only for special occasions or activities such as sports. Such people can switch back to glasses and see well, without the "spectacle blur" associated with hard contact lens wear. Hard contact lenses are so rigid that when worn they tend to round out and make the cornea beneath conform to the shape of the contact lens. For this reason, they can correct astigmatism better, but the cornea shape, having been temporarily altered, is different enough so that glasses worn after removing the contacts do not give consistent vision. This "spectacle blur" means that vision with glasses will vary, depending on how long the contacts have been off. Therefore, there is no such thing as a perfect pair of glasses to wear temporarily for hard contact lens wearers, when not wearing the hard contact lenses. This creates a bit of a problem, because hard contact lens wearers must remove them at bedtime and need backup glasses.

This molding effect of hard lenses has also resulted in a form of treatment of nearsightedness called "orthokeratology," where hard contact lenses are purposely fit flatter than the natural curvature of a patient's cornea, and worn like braces. This flattening results in the feeling of seeing better without glasses for distance than usual, for the nearsighted person, after removing the contact lenses. The lack of success of this treatment is due to variable and imperfect vision, with only temporary results, since the cornea tends to return to its original shape when the contact lenses are not worn. Soft contact lenses, since they conform to the shape of the cornea and are pliable, cause minimal spectacle blur, and thus follow the basic principles of contact lens fitting: not to do any harm or change to the cornea. A pair of glasses may be satisfactory visually, and the patient may switch back and forth between contacts and glasses, when soft contact lenses are chosen.

As mentioned, soft contact lenses are easier and safer than hard contact lenses. Eye doctors now fit mainly soft, daily wear disposable contact lenses, meaning that the lenses are removed at bedtime and replaced about every two weeks. The original soft contact lenses were quite successful, but designed to be worn daily-wear, and replaced every few months. The natural trend was to try to make the lenses last longer, and a syndrome of giant papillary conjunctivitis (GPC) developed. Among the symptoms were that the eye had some irritation, mattering, blurred vision, and the contact lens needed to be replaced more often. Then, when replaced, the new lens did not last long before again demonstrating the symptoms. Examination showed signs of an allergic giant papillary conjunctivitis, whereby flipping or eversion of the upper eyelid showed large papillary growths, so large that the papillae rubbed on the surface of the contact lens so as to destroy the optics and drag the lens upward, as if an eraser was grabbing the lens during blinking. Identification of the syndrome was integral in the development of disposable soft contact lenses. When lenses were worn daily and disposed of in two weeks, the syndrome of GPC became rarely seen, and was recognized as an allergic reaction to the protein buildup on the original soft lenses.

Astigmatism of a significant degree can also be treated also with soft contacts, called toric lenses, but the fitting is more complicated and expensive. It is difficult to obtain as good vision with toric soft contacts as with spectacles or hard contact lenses when dealing with larger degrees of astigmatism. Since specially manufactured to create an astigmatic correction, these toric lenses have a long and short axis of curvature to correct the astigmatism, like a pair of spectacles. However, they must rotate to adjust to the correct axis when first inserted and maintain this position with blinking. Manufacturing specifications make them more expensive to replace, and therefore they are not as disposable as conventional nontoric soft contact lenses.

Safety factors include the fact that soft contact lenses are more fluid and oxygen permeable. Therefore, the "overwear syndrome," commonly seen with hard contact lenses, is relatively unusual with soft contact lenses. The overwear results from lack of oxygen to the cornea that is provided by the normal tears lubricating the cornea. The barrier to these oxygen-providing tears is caused by the relatively oxygen-impermeable hard plastic hard lenses, or even "gas-permeable" hard lenses, which were designed to improve on some of the danger of overwear.

Calls to the eye doctor in the middle of the night have been therefore reduced with the replacement of hard contacts by soft contact lenses. Typically the hard contact lens wearers, usually females, having worn their contact lenses extra long, because of some weekend party or special event, and unaware of any problem, finally removes the contacts and goes to bed. Often air travel is involved. After an interval, the lack of oxygen due to overwear of the contact lenses causes swelling of the cornea and pain so bad that patients are awakened and suspect some more serious problem. If the patients can be made to sleep, with hypnotic or an analgesic, the problem is self-limited, and spontaneously corrected in a matter of hours. In this way, the contact lens overwear syndrome is similar to actinic keratitis (arc welder burn).

Soft contact lens wearers have less chance of overwear, but it can occur, especially with extended wear contacts worn overnight. For this reason, I never suggest extended wear to a beginner. It is too appealing to the "klutzy" person who is too clumsy or scared to handle the lens any more than felt necessary. We want our beginning contact lens wearer to be aware of the dictum that if the eye hurts with the contact lens in, then the contact lens should be removed as the first alternative, and that patients are expected to be confident that they can insert and remove the contact lens anytime wanted. This also means not throwing away old glasses, as they may be needed in such an emergency. However, having demonstrated success at daily wear, extended wear of soft contact lenses may be quite successful in many cases. This of course requires approval and supervision of the eye doctor, since special lenses are designed for extended wear.

There are some other practical things to know about contact lenses. They are more expensive than glasses, but mainly at the beginning. The fitting of contact lenses involves trial fitting, especially with soft lenses, to demonstrate the resulting vision and relative comfort, and then insertion and removal training. Usually this takes about an hour, but sometimes longer. We do not give up on a patient who takes more than one session, since we want them to feel confident. Then there are follow-up visits as needed. Eventually, annual exams are minimally required. Hard or gas-permeable lenses may last for a few years. Disposable soft lenses need to be resupplied usually every six to twelve months. However, the cost of replacing soft contact lenses may be less than that of replacing glasses in the growing child, whose prescription is changing annually.

Cost factors and consumers rights issues have resulted in the fact that eye doctors are "legally" required to give contact lens prescriptions to their patients. However, there are some obvious factors to be clarified. If the patient has never been fitted with contact lenses, then there *is no contact lens prescription.* The eye doctor can guess, but until the patient has been fit successfully with contact lenses, there is no contact lens prescription. Years ago, optical shops that fitted and sold contact lenses were satisfied with the prescription for spectacles and could proceed with the fitting themselves. We told patients that if the contact lens supplier needed more information than their glasses prescription, then "you are in the wrong place." Currently, contact lens "suppliers," such as drugstores or mail order companies, want to merely replace the contact lenses with no responsibility, like selling a shirt, and all they need is the size. This is easier to do with soft contact lenses, which are manufactured to be of identical standards.

Rigid contact lenses are more complicated, and have to be individualized in manufacture, and it is difficult to find a place where these lenses can be replaced other than by the eye doctor. So discount retailers are happy to replace soft contact lenses once they have the prescription. Eye doctors will give the prescription so that patients can get their contact lenses elsewhere, providing that the patient has been successfully fit, and the eye doctor knows what is the successful prescription. Soft contact lenses have the prescription, brand, and size printed on the contact lens package, information needed by a new eye doctor who is expected to give a "prescription" for contact lenses. However, contact lenses obtained elsewhere are not usually under the presumed responsibility of the eye doctor, if there is a problem related to quality of the lenses. And remember, if you have not been successfully fit for contact lenses, meaning that you have paid an eye doctor to satisfactorily fit you, then do not expect an eye doctor to give you "your prescription" for contact lenses. And if you are having problems, and a refit or trial of another kind of contact lens is needed, then be prepared to pay for this service. Once things are again satisfactory to both patient and eye doctor, then the doctor will give you your prescription.

In sports, contact lenses can be a big improvement over glasses. Peripheral vision is better, especially for those with strong prescription spectacles, and the chance of damage to the glasses is eliminated. However, sometimes the contact lens falls out. Whenever you see a basketball or football game stopped to look for a contact lens, however, it usually means the loss of a hard contact lens. Soft contact lenses do not usually fall out or become dislodged with trauma. In some sports, like water polo, an extra large soft lens can be fit to make it even more unlikely that it will be dislodged. However, such a patient would probably have regular soft contact lenses for usual wear. Some urgent care things to know about contact lens complications:

1. If the eye is red or feels uncomfortable, remove the contact lens. A hard contact lens may become quite tight and difficult to remove. In an emergency, it is all right to try something sticky, such as cold marshmallow sundae topping, or cold maple syrup. A dap on the finger will be sticky enough to adhere to the contact lens and help to pull it off. Then the sticky stuff can be rinsed clean from the lens before further use. A soft contact lens is usually removed differently, but it also could be removed by such a sticky substance, the difference being that the lens would have to be thrown away. One of the potential problems, especially in soft contact lens wear, is the fact that the lens may have already come off, and attempts to remove a contact lens no longer

in place may be irritating to the eye. One should be able to test the vision, and if it is fairly normal, then the contact lens may still be in place. If the vision is poor, similar to when the lens is off, then the contact lens is probably no longer in place. By the way, do not worry about the lens going behind the eye; it cannot. It may hide under the upper eyelid if a hard lens, but most soft lenses are large enough so that there is not enough room to hide under the lid.

2. If one or both eyes are chronically red, not comfortable, and light sensitive, then whether one wears hard or soft contact lenses, they should not be worn, and exam by your regular eye doctor is indicated.

3. Appearance of a white spot on the cornea, over the colored, iris part of the eye, may indicate a corneal irritation from contact lens wear, hard or soft. Sometimes such a problem is called an "ulcer," signifying a more serious problem, but usually the problem is due to lack of oxygen, and can be treated without serious scarring. Certainly it is not something to ignore.

4. Overwear of a contact lens results in oxygen deprivation to the cornea, and the resultant pain is often within an interval of a few hours after the lens is removed, and is therefore confusing about the cause. A hard or gas-permeable lens should not be worn overnight, for example, and overwear may result from even a little increase in wear over routine, or aggravated by air travel, or bright sunlight, as in sunbathing. Usually the symptoms are greatly improved by time and topical steroid drops, after removing the contact lens. Soft contact lenses are safer in general as to overwear, but certainly, sleeping with a daily wear contact lens in place, or wearing an extended wear contact lens too long, can result in discomfort and blurred vision, at least temporarily.

5. Air travel for the contact lens wearer can be a problem. With hard lenses especially, the time in air travel can lead to symptoms of overwear sooner than expected. I suggest that if hard contact lens wearers are expecting a need to wear the lenses longer than usual, they take a break for a few hours during the day, in order to get away with wearing the lenses until later at night, as for a big party. Dryness can create a problem even for the soft contact lens wearers, so that lubricating drops are indicated.

6. Yes, you can get green soft contact lenses, as well as other colors available to alter your eye color. These are even available in prescription powers. However, plano (lenses without prescription power) cosmetic contact lens wear has been restricted legally to avoid indiscriminate wear by untrained persons, and the trading off of lenses from one person to another, usually a teenager, with the subsequent risk of spreading eye infection or eye injury. Hard contact lenses are usually tinted slightly in order to make them easier to find and handle, but not enough to change eye color. Since they are smaller, blue lenses on brown eyes would look weird.

7. Recently there has been concern about several cases of a rare fungus infection known as fusarium keratitis. Coincidental connection with a common contact lens cleaning solutic.. resulted in the company's withdrawing the solution from distribution, though information was not complete enough to make a certain connection. Such cases call to attention that there is potential for infection among contact lens wearers, and it is actually amazing that the incidence of infection is so low. It is recommended to wash hands with soap and water

and then dry them before handling the lenses. The lenses should be regularly cleaned by rubbing and rinsing, replaced at regular recommended intervals, and stored in a clean, dry case that is replaced every three to six months. At least times have changed since the old-timer hard contact lens wearers felt that some of their own spit provided the best lubrication for inserting their lenses.

5

VISUAL ACUITY

Before we get more into reading glasses, refractive surgery, eye disease, cataract surgery, and so forth, maybe we should talk about what we are trying to preserve: good vision.

What is normal vision? We speak of 20/20 as the standard. What does that mean? Well, in a rather basic sense, it means you can see at 20 feet what you should see at 20 feet. In metric terms, one can see at 6 meters what one should see at 6 meters. Similarly, 20/40 vision, means you see at 20 feet, what you should be able to see at 40 feet, if things were normalized. This is the level of vision required to obtain a driver's license in most states; in other words, not perfect, but pretty good vision. Then there is the reference to uncorrected and corrected vision. What is most important is how good one can see, even if glasses are required, as in "corrected vision." Too often, emphasis is placed on uncorrected vision, or how well one sees without glasses. This is where there is often extreme confusion as to what is meant by "legal blindness." This statement is frequently used incorrectly, such as saying someone was "legally blind" before refractive surgery, when actually this is not true at all. Shame on any eye doctors who advertise this way. Legal blindness means 20/200 vision or worse, *even with* glasses, or corrected vision. Many nearsighted people cannot see the 20/200 letters on the eye chart without glasses, but with glasses they usually see 20/20. And they can often see 20/20 up close without glasses. Legal blindness means no better than 20/200 vision even with correction (glasses), *at any distance.* Too often, the result of refractive or cataract surgery is advertised in reference to unaided vision at distance. However, a so-called good result of uncorrected vision may actually result in imperfect vision with best correction. So a person may be happy to see better without glasses, but the best result would be also no loss of vision with best correction.

Passing a driver's license visual requirement is of utmost importance to most adults. People also do not want to be restricted to wearing glasses for driving. Most nearsighted persons expect to be told they need glasses for driving, but many others, either because they have not had an eye exam, or because they used to see well without glasses, are quite surprised to be told they need to have glasses for driving. My advise for those who think they can pass is to go ahead and take the test without glasses. If they pass, fine. But if they fail, then pull out the prescription glasses and pass. Then, of course because of better vision with glasses, the license will say that glasses must be worn. So then you better get used to wearing your glasses, so that if you are ever pulled over in a traffic stop, you can avoid a ticket by having your glasses on. However, if you fail even with glasses and have been told by your eye doctor that you should pass, ask for the form for your doctor to fill out. I recall one patient to whom I told this, and she later called saying that I had told her to call if she failed the DMV test. I said, "So you flunked the eye test," and she said, "No, I flunked the written." I had to tell her I could not do anything about that.

Loss of a driver's license is often extremely devastating to the elderly, as Dr. Robert Levine points out in his book *Aging with Attitude.* The number of people considered elderly is increasing rapidly and represents a large percentage of the population in some states. Some states make testing procedures more frequent or intense for the elderly, which may not seem fair, but then problems that could affect safe driving are increasingly common as we get older, and much of this can be due to poor uncorrected or corrected vision. Loss of the driver's license means loss of status and independence for the elderly, and for many it signifies the beginning of the end. There is a gender (macho) effect in this problem, because it is very difficult for a husband to give away the driving rights to his wife; I mean he has to be really seeing badly before he will give up the wheel. But then there is the story about the ninety-four-year-old man in assisted living, who tells his buddy that he is getting married. His friend questions why to get married at his age:" Is this woman real pretty?" "No, she is ninety, so what would you guess?" "Well, is she rich?" "No, she doesn't have much money." "Well then, can she cook?" "No, she can't cook worth a lick." "Well then, why are you marrying her?" "Well, she can drive, and *at night.*"

One-eyed people are naturally concerned about passing a driver's test, but usually only one good seeing eye is required for a license. Routinely, this means that your eye doctor will need to fill out a form stating why you only see well with one eye, even with glasses. If the worse eye can be made to see well with glasses, you may be required to wear glasses for driving, but your eye doctor can ask for an exception if it is determined that wearing the glasses would be confusing. This may be true if a person has anisometropia, a marked difference between the eyes, whereby wearing glasses may not improve the second-best eye to normal, and may cause confusion due to difference in image sizes. Once the eye doctor fills out the form, a person may be required to have the form filled out every time the license is to be renewed, and unfortunately the license may be only for one year at a time. Motor vehicle department clerks do not know much about eye conditions, and may tend to be "officious" about details involving forms. And let's face it, the form they work with is antiquated and unworkable in many cases.

Is there such a thing as supernormal vision, and how can it be obtained? Well, the incidence of better than 20/20 vision is quite high, with or without glasses—20/15 or even 20/10 vision is not unusual. The ability to see this well is innate, but may require glasses. There is no treatment to improve vision. Athletes such as Ted Williams do not have supernormal vision, their visual performances probably being best explained by exceptional concentration ability and eye-hand coordination, which are perhaps not teachable. If a person is able to see no better than 20/20 with correction, then cataract or refractive surgery cannot expect to make vision any better than that. Exercises and alternative medicines may be advertised as improving vision. Can exercises change the shape of the eye, or make an eye see better than it ever potentially did? The answer is no, of course not.

Exercises cannot change the shape of the eye. They cannot make you no longer nearsighted. However, the idea of improving vision with exercises has hung around for a long time, first popularized by Dr. W.H. Bates, who wrote a book in 1920. Though a study refuted his anecdotal claims, others have persisted in "selling" such notions for profit. More recently, the "See Clearly Method" has attracted much advertising attention, and also, I understand, the attention of antifraud action.

Focusing problems may seem to be something possibly helped by corrective exercises. However, the measure of reading ability is quite subjective, often even in a testing situation, making results of things such as focusing training difficult to objectively measure. Certainly, one's ability to read with or without glasses is affected by such things as lighting, state of rest, size of pupil, size of print, contrast of print as in soft- versus hardcover books, and variations of black on white print of various newspapers. Therefore, if you have reading glasses, it is more objective to rate your vision on the basis of how you see with the corrective glasses, rather than be concerned about apparent variations of vision without glasses. Also, according to the best information, focusing problems are not secondary to "weak muscles," but are rather due to the increasing rigidity of the normal lens of the eye with age, making focusing efforts less successful. Therefore, exercises expected to "strengthen" the focusing muscles of the eye are not expected to be help.

PART II

COMMON EYE PROBLEMS

6

EVERYDAY MALADIES

There are many reasons to want to see an eye doctor other than routine eye exams to test vision. Some are emergencies, but, if one understands some basics about the eyes, the need to seek care can be recognized as urgent or not so urgent. Some understanding of eye problems, however, cannot replace actually seeing the eye doctor.

THE RED EYE

There are many causes of red eyes, and here are some of the more common.

Pink Eye (Conjunctivitis)

This is a common infection affecting one or both eyes, and the conjunctiva, the thin outermost vascular layer of tissue covering the white of the eye. It can occur at any age, but is most common in schoolchildren, who can then infect siblings and parents. There are basically two kinds, viral and bacterial. Viral conjunctivitis does not respond to antibiotics and may accompany an upper respiratory infection (a cold). Corneal involvement may occur with viral infections, causing foreign body sensation, blurred vision, and photophobia. The average duration is two weeks, and, as mentioned, antibiotics do not cure, but, in some situations, antibiotic-steroid combinations may lessen discomfort. Bacterial conjunctivitis usually has a more purulent discharge than viral infections and will respond to antibiotic eye drops, sometimes promptly. Although experienced eye doctors can sometimes tell viral from bacterial infections, they often cannot be sure, either, until following the course of the infection. Both types are contagious, and share the fact that the second eye is usually less severely affected. Viral contagion may be actually "epidemic" in spread, so that schoolchildren should not return to school until recovered. Caregivers (parents) should be careful to wash their hands after applying eye drops to their children patients.

Spontaneous Conjunctival Hemorrhage

This is another kind of red eye, which may appear quite serious, because the eye is so red. However, the redness is localized, usually to part of one eye, and looks worse than it really is. Spontaneous bleeding from a conjunctival vessel can occur for unknown reasons, the usual story being that a person wakes up, looks in the mirror, and there it is. There is no pain, no discharge, and no blurred vision. If one is taking anticoagulants, the incidence is more common, but usually it is a spontaneous problem without any health significance. Of course, trauma to the eye or periorbital tissue can cause this form of bruising, which is associated with a "black eye." The downside is that there is no treatment, since the blood has to absorb like a bruise, becoming yellowish as it absorbs. The biggest complication is having to reassure everyone who sees you that it is not as bad as it seems, and that if you did see the doctor, he could not do anything to make it go away. Wearing sunglasses can help avoid unwanted attention.

Episcleritis

This is usually more of a localized redness of one eye, without discharge, but also usually more uncomfortable in terms of pain. It is not an infection, so it is not contagious, and vision is usually not affected. The tissue deeper than the superficial conjunctiva is involved, but it is sometimes difficult to tell the difference from conjunctivitis by appearance alone. The cause is relatively unknown, but it can be associated with inflammatory conditions such as arthritis. It is usually unilateral, but can recur in the same or other eye. The treatment is to use topical steroid drops, rarely oral steroids, but not antibiotics. Response can be prompt or delayed.

Iritis (Iridocyclitis)

Such inflammation may be indicated by a localized redness of the eye, the redness being a ring around the pupil tissue, the colored part of the eye. However, it may be generalized, especially in more severe cases. The pupil becomes smaller, and since usually monocular, the pupil of the red eye is smaller compared with that of the other eye. The diagnosis requires microscopic or "slit lamp" confirmation, with which "flare" (increased protein in the chamber in front of the pupil) and cells (white blood cells visible in the same area) can be identified. Since the pupil tissue (iris) is inflamed, it become sticky, and may stick to the front surface of the lens, causing scar tissue that can affect the roundness of the pupil. Also, because the pupil tissue is involved, sensitivity to light is a prime symptom.

Localized redness, with photophobia, and small pupil would be thought to make the diagnosis easy, but iritis is too often mistaken for conjunctivitis. The treatment involves steroid eye drops, dilating the pupil, and in severe cases, use of oral steroids. Iritis is often primary, involving only one eye, but can be secondary, as resulting from injury or irritation of the cornea. However, it also can be recurrent and affect the same or other eye. It is rarely bilateral, and the cause is usually unknown, but the tendency can accompany inflammatory arthritic conditions, such as ankylosing spondylitis. The relationship may be recognized, but iritis is not necessarily found parallel to symptomatic recurrence of arthritis.

Though the pupil may become scarred, vision is rarely affected, when the iritis is treated properly. Paradoxically, dilating the affected pupil, instead of making the photophobia worse by letting more light in, causes relief by putting the pupil to rest. This allows the other eye to be not bothered by light, since both pupils normally work together in reaction to light, or in reading. By putting the inflamed pupil to rest, the reaction of the noninflamed eye to light or reading will not cause pain in the inflamed eye. As with other inflammatory ocular conditions of unknown cause, such as episcleritis, recurrences become less common with age—one of the rare advantages of getting older.

Scleritis

It is rather uncommon and is a deeper-layer inflammation than episcleritis, inflammation of the white of the eye itself. The redness is also localized, but the pain is quite intense, enough to suggest urgent care. The treatment is topical and oral corticosteroids, and requires close follow-up by an ophthalmologist.

Acute Angle Closure Glaucoma

It causes a red eye (rarely bilateral) and is accompanied by pain in the eyebrow, blurred vision, pupil enlargement, and a rapid rise in intraocular pressure. Nausea and vomiting may occur, thus obscuring the source of the problem. Treatment is one of the eye emergencies, and is discussed as a form of glaucoma in Chapter 11.

FOREIGN BODY SENSATION ("SOMETHING IN THE EYE")

Corneal Foreign Body

It is most common, as objects can enter the eye with such force as to stick or become imbedded into the superficial cornea. A corneal foreign body causes sensation of something under the upper eyelid, and patients often need reassurance that removing the corneal object is the correct treatment. Metallic foreign bodies are common, especially in those who use drilling or cutting tools. Ferrous (iron) foreign bodies cause a telltale rust buildup in a matter of hours, so that removal of the foreign body may be easier than that of the resultant "rust ring." If centrally located, a large rust ring can leave a scar that may affect vision. The removal is usually best performed with a "spud," or a similar sharp-tipped instrument, and is best accomplished with aid of a slit lamp (microscope). The eye can be anesthetized easily, as topical anesthesia works very well on the cornea. Patients need reassurance about this.

Conjunctival Foreign Body

This is less painful, depending on the size and location of the particle. If located inside the lower eyelid, the object may actually work out spontaneously or rise to the corner of the eye, where it can be seen and wiped away with a cotton swab. If located under the upper eyelid, it may cause significant discomfort until removed. This may require eversion, or flipping of the upper eyelid, so as to expose the inside surface where such foreign bodies can be trapped and cause scratching of the cornea. Relief is prompt, so that concern for additional foreign bodies is relieved. If there is still any doubt about remaining foreign bodies, it is wise to irrigate the eye with water if special irrigating fluids are not available. There need not be concern that a foreign body may work its way behind the eye; it can only go a few millimeters under the eyelid. If the foreign body scratches the cornea, then there may be some residual foreign body sensation, of a lesser degree, after removal of the foreign body, until the scratch heals in a few hours. Artificial lubricating tears would be soothing until healing is completed.

Eversion or flipping the upper eyelid is something that is done by the eye doctor, but is also something possibly discoverable by young people, usually as a joke. However, when the upper lid is everted, or flipped, there are some bulges that may make a person concerned about a mass pressing on the eye. I have seen more than one patient for this reason, thinking that there is some sort of tumor of the eyelid; one was a son of a local dentist. The upper eyelid has a cartilage-like tissue in the center, the tarsus, which conforms to the roundness of the eyeball in the usual position, but if flipped, it causes a bulge toward the nose and toward the ear.

Trichiasis

Trichiasis, or the in-turning of an eyelash, can cause foreign body sensation. The lash may be so small as to be difficult to see with the naked eye, and certainly difficult to remove without professional help. Epilation, or removal of the offending eyelash, gives immediate relief. Unfortunately, eyelashes that grow in a crooked direction may regrow, again in the same direction and require repeated epilation. To prevent regrowth, cautery units are available to try to destroy the germinal origin of the lash.

Corneal Abrasion, or Scratched Cornea

This injury can cause foreign body sensation of a mild to severe degree, depending on how much of the epithelium, or surface layer, of the cornea is damaged. The cornea, the window transparent tissue over the pupil, is the most sensitive tissue in the body. A scratch can occur from many causes, including the probing finger of an infant. It is usually so small as to be invisible to the naked eye, but the feeling as if something is in the eye, or under the upper eyelid, is present until the abrasion is healed. Fortunately, healing occurs rapidly but sometimes needs encouragement. Patching of the eye controls blinking and thus encourages healing. In some cases a bandage contact lens may speed return to usual activity. Prescription eye drops may be needed, and even artificial tears may soothe the cornea while healing.

Keratitis

Keratitis, or any inflammation of the cornea, can cause foreign body sensation. This can accompany conjunctivitis of a viral variety, be associated with dry eye or contact lens wear, injury such as in a scratched cornea, or anything that disturbs the healthy surface contour of the cornea. Microscopic exam by an eye doctor is usually required to make the diagnosis before initiating treatment. However, sometimes such an abrasion can be seen with a flourescein stain, without magnification. Significant corneal irritation is accompanied by photophobia, which is a sign of at least mild secondary iritis. Actinic keratitis is due to ultraviolet exposure and results in swelling of the cornea to the point where severe pain results. It will be discussed more in chapter eighteen.

Recurrent Corneal Erosion

This is a condition whereby the sensation of something in the eye recurs, mildly or sometimes quite painfully. Typically, the problem originates upon awakening in the morning and may be so transient that later in the day the sensation of foreign body is gone. Then the problem may recur and last longer or be more severe. Topical lubricants, such as ointments, at bedtime or daytime artificial tears may give relief, at least temporarily. A more severe episode may require patching or bandage contact lens. Examination shows an area of the corneal epithelium, the superficial layer, which does not heal properly, and may show evidence between attacks upon microscopic examination with a slit lamp. The problem seems to be a defect in the usual healing ability of the surface cells, the epithelium of the cornea. These cells can be likened to bricks in a brick wall, which are held together by mortar. The epithelium cells can normally regenerate or heal quite rapidly, in a matter of hours. However, in the case of recurrent corneal erosion, it is as if the material that holds the cells together, the mortarlike intercellular substance, is defective. Thus, the slightest trauma, perhaps even a blink, causes the cells to flake off, like bricks crumbling from a wall, and causes irritation of the pain sensation nerves. Treatment can involve eye drops containing antibiotic-steroids, ointments and lubricating drops, patching or bandage contact lenses, and sometimes minor surgical procedures to encourage better healing. The original cause is usually obscure, but may have been from a scratched cornea, or even spontaneous in onset.

HERPETIC OCULAR DISEASE

Herpes Simple Virus (Cold Sore Virus)

This virus causes keratoconjunctivitis, which can be commonly unrecognized as due to herpes simplex type I. The biggest problem in recognition of this specific type virus is that it can appear to be something else, such as a regular pink eye. It is sometimes called the great masquerader, because even for an eye doctor it can be difficult to diagnose. If traditional, it causes a "dendritic figure" type of corneal infiltrate, which is too microscopic to detect with the naked eye. The cornea also tends to be relatively numb.

The difficulty in recognizing this viral infection is mainly responsible for the caution for nonophthalmic doctors to never use a topical steroid eye drop in treating apparent eye inflammation. This is because use of topical steroids may worsen or prolong recovery from herpes infection. Paradoxically, topical steroids may be indicated if herpetic disease becomes deeper, involving the "stroma" of the cornea. Nevertheless, this is a decision left to the ophthalmologist.

For the antiviral treatment of herpes simplex virus (HSV), topical eye drops such as Viroptic, or a similar ointment, are used, and positive results can usually be seen within a few days. However, the medication is irritating to the eye and needs to be titrated so as to not prolong illness. The usual antibiotic eye drops do not work, but it is better for the non-eye doctor to stick to such medication when the cause is unknown, before the patient is seen by an eye doctor. An oral antiviral such as Acyclovir is also sometimes used, whether really necessary or not, because it has such few side effects and will at least do no harm.

Other than the common misdiagnosis of HSV I, the most important thing to remember is that it can recur, without obvious cause other than a minor ocular trauma. Like a cold sore, it recurs in the same place, such as on the lip (labial HSV). The history of HSV infection should always be made known to anyone treating this same eye in the future. It is rare to involve the other eye primarily or secondarily.

HSV II is the sexually transmitted form of the infection, and involves the genitalia. Its spread to the eye would be rare and by mechanical transfer. It is also possible to transfer HSV I by inoculation, for example, a mother with a labial infection kissing the face of her infant. This would ordinarily result in an eyelid, infection, not corneal infection, and be accompanied by a large pre-auricular lymph node (gland in front of the ear).

Primary herpes blepharitis is also possible because of HSV I. It causes a blisterlike lesion localized to a portion of the eyelid and responds to antiviral ointment. Recurrence in the same place is sometimes a later confirmation of diagnosis.

Herpes Zoster Virus (HZV)

This infection causes shingles, which is supposedly the same as the chicken pox virus, and can involve the eyes. After recovering from chickenpox, the virus remains alive in the patient but inactive in certain nerve roots for years. It commonly involves the nerves around the ribs, and around the eye it can involve branches of the facial nerve. Most commonly involved is the ophthalmic branch of the trigeminal nerve, with the first symptoms being a vesicular (blisterlike) eruption in the area served by this nerve branch. Such skin lesions can therefore go from forehead up into the hairline, but just on one side of the head, and specifically not crossing the midline. The skin lesions heal, often rapidly enough that the scalp needs to be examined to help make the diagnosis.

Skin involvement may vary; and the skin may only involve only small areas, for example, only the inner part of the upper eyelid. Typically, if the tip of the nose is involved, the eyeball itself will likely be also. However, eye involvement should be suspected with any form of shingles around the eye. The eye may develop only a mild conjunctivitis, but if the cornea is involved there can be lasting, even severe, complications. There can be various kinds of keratitis, even appearing like HSV I, but the more severe involvement is intraocular, when it occurs, in the form of iridocyclitis of varying degree.

Treatment involves topical steroid drops, dilating drops if there is iritis, and oral Acyclovir antiviral medication if indicated. Iris atrophy with pupil distortion may result, but eventually the process clears. Unfortunately, there are recurrences, and long-term maintenance medication may be required. A new development is the recommendation for those over age sixty to be vaccinated with a new drug called Zostavax as a means of prevention, since the older one gets, the greater are the chances of developing shingles, reaching 50 percent over age eighty-five.

LACRIMAL DISORDERS

Dry Eye (Keratoconjunctivitis Sicca)

This is a very common problem, to variable degree. Tears are natural lubrication fluids formed by conjunctival glands and the lacrimal gland. Confusion surrounds discussion of the tear duct, which actually drains fluid from the eyes, down the nose; hence the nose "runs" when one cries. Some are confused into thinking that the tear duct caries tears from the tear gland. Tear formation is relatively constant from conjunctival glands, but can be affected by diseases of the conjunctiva. The lacrimal gland is relatively large, is located laterally and superiorly in the upper eyelid, and functions reflexively to irritation and emotion. Dry eye is usually due to inadequate tear production by the conjunctival glands. When associated with rheumatoid arthritis, the dry eye is part of Sjögren's syndrome. Improper tear lubrication can be likened to trying to see through a car windshield when the window wiper or washer does not clear the view. Mucous shreds make the tear film sticky, so that the normal blink can just smear things around, like bugs resisting the effect of the windshield wiper. Blinking may also be defective, as for example in Bell's Palsy. Symptoms may be worse when reading or using a computer, because of decreased blinking. Air conditioners or heaters can cause drying because of the increased evaporation of tears, so that people may be more uncomfortable after a trip in the car. Air travel is especially drying to the eyes.

Most dry eye problems are spontaneous and perhaps more common in women. In addition to health problems such as rheumatoid arthritis, the wearing of contact lenses, even soft ones, may cause dry eyes. Dry eyes are also a complication of lasik refractive surgery, on a temporary or prolonged basis.

Treatment involves tear supplements, in the form of artificial tears, which are available without prescription. Plugging the tear duct opening, the punctum, may be necessary in severe cases, either temporarily or permanently. However, those wanting a "quick fix," or those who have heard of such a treatment, sometimes come into the office demanding such treatment, without realizing that it can cause unwanted watering of the eyes. Some newer eye drops, containing cyclosporin (Restasis), offer hope of more permanent help, though treatment results can be delayed until treated a long time, and may be more effective in females than males. Because of "direct advertising," you will hear a lot about Restasis. However, if you read the small print in the package insert, you will find that the improvement results of a study group showed that after 6 months of use by a large study group 15 percent improved tear production, after having used Restasis for six months compared with 5 percent who used other treatment, as demonstrated by the "Schirmer's" test, a measuring test for tear production. Supporters point out that this study was performed on severe cases of dry eyes, and claim that those with less severe problems may achieve higher success.

As mentioned, lasik surgery can cause dry eyes. Some lasik surgeons routinely place punctual plugs after the lasik, as if it is for sure that there will be a dry eye problem. True, this may be helpful, if the eyes are dry, but maybe it is to shortcut any complaints, since the refractive surgeon does not want to be involved in postoperative care. What if watering of the eyes occurs eventually. Guess then the plugs should be removed, but does the patient know about all this? And who is supposed to do this? There can be a lack of communication, as I have observed.

Tearing (Epiphora)

Tearing is also common and can be more common with increasing age. However, congenital tearing problems are also frequent, but these usually spontaneously improve. Probing the tear duct may be necessary in infants, but is less successful in adults in cases of acquired tear duct obstruction. Treatment of congenital lacrimal obstruction has varied in intensity through the years, the main attention now being toward treating the lacrimal tract infection until the mattering and tearing improve.

Inflammation may be a cause of swelling of the tear duct or tear sac (a reservoir for tear collection), in children or adults, so that antibiotic eye drops or oral antibiotics may be needed to correct the problem. The tear sac is located where the upper and lower lids come together, in the inner "canthus." When swollen, it is a palpable and sometimes visible bulge in this area. When infected, this bulge can be tender, and pressure may cause regurgitation of mucopurulent material out of the punctum.

Sometimes, a new opening needs to be made into the nose surgically, called dacryocystorhinostomy, but this can usually be avoided. Eyelid abnormalities can contribute to the tearing problem, such as drooping of the lower lid outward (ectropian), or improper blinking as in Bell's palsy. It is of some comfort to understand that tearing to some degree is commonly acquired and is certainly preferable to lack of tears, as in dry eyes. My personal experience is that I have never seen an adult patient with tearing dating to childhood, which suggests that spontaneous improvement is certainly the rule. (Questioning colleagues has given the same impression.)

SPOTS IN VISION

Floaters and Flashes

Spots in vision, which move with the movement of the eye in a floating manner, are called floaters. These are quite common, especially noted against a light blue sky, and represent a minor nuisance. The sudden onset of a large floater, of various size or shape, is frequently accompanied by a sensation of light flashes, especially at night and with movement of the eye. These are symptoms of what is called a vitreous detachment. The vitreous is a jellylike fluid that mainly consists of a waterlike fluid, but is gel-like in consistency, and occupies most of the space behind the lens of the eye. It can become more liquid and shift about, so as to exert traction on the retina. A loose attachment around the optic nerve can pull away, causing a rather large floater, which can be noted to be oval or round, but can appear any shape. The sloshing around of the vitreous gel can create the sensation of light flashes, since the retina recognizes most stimuli as light sensation. The light flashes stop in a matter of days or weeks, as if the retina gets used to the sensation.

Usually, there is no serious consequence, but the onset of floaters and flashes, or even just large floaters, should indicate the need to be examined by an eye doctor. This is because these symptoms may be the first sign of a retinal detachment, a serious condition that sometimes needs emergency treatment, often surgical. If a careful retinal exam shows no sign of retinal hole or detachment, then there is no need for restriction of activity and generally no need to worry. However, a recurrence of new floaters, especially a "shower" of floaters, which could mean bleeding inside the vitreous, or a shadow coming from the side vision that does not go away, should stimulate prompt return to your ophthalmologist to look for a retinal detachment.

The vitreous floater or floaters, unfortunately, may persist for an indefinite time. The question is asked whether they can be removed. Technically, they can, by surgical vitrectomy, but the cost and potential complications make this an unreasonable option. Actually, in almost all cases, the floaters cease to be a problem, even if under certain circumstances, such as against a blue sky, the floaters may reappear transiently. There seems to be a combination of "getting used to it" and the movement of the symptom, causing materials out of the line of sight. Also, perhaps, some may absorb or somehow disintegrate.

Stationary Spots

A spot in the vision, usually centrally, which does not float or move, but seems stationary, may be something more significant, especially if associated with vision loss. Eye exam may show a swelling of the macula (as in central serous retinopathy or diabetic macular edema), or hemorrhage in the macula (as in vascular occlusion, macular degeneration, or diabetic retinopathy). Vision is usually reduced, and an Amsler grid or visual field examination may show signs of central scotoma (blackout of vision centrally).

Ocular Migraine

Episodic spots in the vision, along with other assorted weird visual sensations, can be due to a common problem called ophthalmic migraine. Such episodes usually last 15–30 minutes, though descriptions vary. A typical episode starts with the sensation of having looked at something too bright, causing the sensation of seeing spots similar to being dazzled by a big flash camera. Because of this, many will swear that looking at a light caused the episode (and sometimes don't want a light shined in their eyes for examination). The next phase involves sensations of seeing flashing lights, zigzag lines, heat wave effects, or looking through water, or a TV out of focus, and is usually the phase that most people recall most vividly. The final phase, which is sometimes not recognized by people, is blacking out of half of the vision, everything to the right or left. Because of this, they will sometimes think that either the right or the left eye is involved, depending on which side experiences the loss of vision toward the ear, the bigger "half" of side vision.

When informed of the connection to migraine, many refuse to believe this, since they often have no headache. If there is no headache, then the syndrome is called ocular or ophthalmic migraine. The onset may be later in life and is more common in women, the trigger mechanism being hormone level fluctuation, and can occur even if hormones are being taken (HRT). There is no treatment, other than treating hormonal irregularities, if needed, since the episodes are very brief, and usually infrequent. Well, beta-blockers would probably avoid such episodes, but most would not like the side effects. However, with warning signs of an attack, one should pull over for a while when driving a car, because the vision will be affected for a few minutes. The trigger mechanism in men is less clear, but it may be due to women (smile).

However, it is known that preservatives in food or wine are the cause in some (e.g. hot dogs).

If a headache occurs, it follows the visual prodrome, and then the problem is called "classical migraine." Compared with most migraine headaches, which are often severe and associated with nausea and vomiting, the headache may be mild and usually on one side of the head.

LUMPS AND BUMPS OF THE EYES

Tender Bumps on the Eyelids

These are usually due to a stye (hordeolum). They are similar to pimples or boils elsewhere on the body, and are caused by infection of an eyelid gland with staphylococcus, the common skin pathogen bacteria. Treatment can include hot compresses to bring the lesion to a "head" so that it can pop and drain spontaneously. Topical antibiotics are also used, and rarely are oral antibiotics necessary. Surgical drainage is not usually necessary, or even preferred, since premature attempt to drain the sty may cause unnecessary spread of the infection.

Cysts of the Eyelid (Chalazia)

A chalazion may start out somewhat tender, like a stye, but the tenderness lessens and a cyst containing cottage cheesy stuff develops. It does not drain spontaneously, since the contents are thicker than pus, and may continue to enlarge. If small, it may spontaneously go away, absorbing gradually. If larger, it may need to be drained, in the doctor's office usually. Those located in the upper eyelid may press internally on to the eye, so as to rub on the cornea or blur vision, and therefore need drainage even though not large. If the occurrence of chalazia is frequent, then tetracycline oral medication may be needed, much like a person with acne sometimes needs. Tiny white-head-like cysts or clear-fluid-containing cysts may occur on the eyelid margins, but neither usually of significant need for treatment.

Pterygium

This is a small growth originating in the conjunctiva, usually toward the nose, which grows onto the cornea. Most pterygia stop growing spontaneously, but some grow over to block the pupil, unless surgically removed. Complicating the decision about treatment is the fact that the eye easily becomes very red, so that cosmetically it is a problem. If the redness can be minimized, it becomes less of a problem, as the growth eventually becomes inactive. Use of decongestants to "take the red out" needs be limited, because the rebound effect may make the redness worse. Another problem is that surgically removing the pterygium may be followed with about 50 percent recurrence rate, sometimes even to a worse degree, unless something like beta irradiation is used to lessen the recurrence. Most people are reassured to know that the growth is likely to be very slow, so that one can take time considering treatment alternatives. The number of surgical approaches to recurrences helps prove that there is no guaranteed treatment. The cosmetic problems become less in time, so that patience to allow the pterygium to become inactive and stop growing seems advisable in most cases.

Pingueculum

This is another small growth on the conjunctiva, usually toward the nose, but may also originate toward the ear. It is usually slightly yellow, and represents a thickening surrounded by extra blood vessels. It may not be noticeable, unless the eye is irritated. Then it becomes thicker and the surrounding blood vessels dilate, making the eye look red. With time, a pingueculum will also become thinner and less noticeable. Removal is not recommended, because usually it is not necessary and because the lesion may grow back more active, and even develop into a pterygium.

Tumors of the Eyelid

These may be benign or malignant. Basal cell carcinomas and squamous carcinomas may occur, and can often be identified as to type with the slit lamp microscope. The eyelid margin is frequently the site, so that removal is more complicated. The tumor cannot just be superficially cut away without leaving a notch or defect in the lid margin that would not allow protection of the cornea. Also, usual techniques of wide excision must be minimized, and frozen section pathology techniques may be utilized to ensure that the tumor has been completely removed. After tumor removal, the defect must be closed by careful realignment of the lid tissues, so as to reform the lid margin and return the lid to as normal a functioning as possible. Usually this can be done if the tumor is not allowed to become too large.

Nevus of the eyelid is also common. Though benign, those which involve the lid margin are not so simple to remove, for the same reasons as malignant tumors present. Shaving it off leaves deeper roots that will cause recurrence. The nevus must be wedged out, and full thickness repair is involved to avoid notching of the eyelid. With this in mind, and because a nevus can be expected to become minimal in full size, it is usually advisable to observe the nevus and plan to not remove it unless it becomes significantly large. Removal of lid margin tumors, benign or malignant, are best managed by an ophthalmic plastic surgeon rather than a dermatologist or general plastic surgeon.

EYELID DISORDERS

Ectropion

This is a drooping down of the lower lid. It can be along the entire length of the lower eyelid or confined to the part near the nose, which means that the tear duct is involved and tearing is a problem. The usual cause is the unfortunate complication of sagging of facial tissues with age. It can also be a complication following a face-lift, whereby extra or sagging skin is removed, and the face "tightened up." This, of course, means that too much skin has been removed, and if it occurs early following surgery, it may get a bit better as the skin is allowed to stretch some more. When tearing is involved, people tend to rub their eyes or dab at them to blot the tears away. Unfortunately, this tends to make to ectropion worse. Treatment is usually surgical, involving pulling the lid laterally to suspend it, and sometimes a skin graft. When the ectropion is mainly toward the nose, involving the tear duct opening, the punctum, it is rather difficult to fix, and if not a big cosmetic problem, it may be best left untreated.

Entropion

This is an inward turning of the eyelid, usually the lower eyelid. Having to do with tissue laxity, it too occurs more in the elder population. For example, it may be the cause of chronic mattering in the eye of a nursing home patient. Sometimes this problem is not obvious, because the eyelid appears to be in position. However, close inspection demonstrates that the eyelashes are not visible. Gentle traction on the lower lid allows the eyelash row to pop back into view, often with relief of the scratchy sensation caused by the eyelashes rubbing against the conjunctiva. However, the relief is usually transient, as the eyelid flips back inward, often with just a blink. Another problem is that the irritation caused by the in-turned eyelashes causes one to often close the eyes tightly, which makes the condition worse because forced closure triggers the flipping inward of the lower lid. Temporary treatment can involve taping to help keep the lid pulled out. Sometimes a special suturing technique works, but a more permanent result may require special surgery, with the careful shifting of lid structures. Surgical overcorrection could cause the opposite problem, ectropion.

Blepharitis

This is probably the most common eyelid problem and represents a usually chronic condition of inflammation of the glands of the eyelid (meibomian glands) and eyelash follicles. Commonly, it is part of generalized skin condition such as seborrheic dermatitis, but may also be associated with psoriasis or rosacea. Hypersensitivity to staphylococcus, the common bacterium contaminant of the skin, is often a factor. Signs of the problem include redness along the eyelid margin, crusts on the eyelashes, and frequent styes or chalazia. Treatment is usually a long-term process, including eyelid hygiene involving cleaning crusts from the eyelashes, and when significant, use of antibiotic or antibiotic/steroid, ointment, or drops for intervals of time. Those who have seborrheic tendencies should treat their scalp seborrhea, and avoid hairstyles involving "bangs" hanging over the eyebrows. Frequent associated styes or chalazia may suggest interval use of oral tetracyclines.

Ptosis

This is a drooping of the upper eyelid, making the eye appear smaller, and limiting the aperture, or space, between the eyelids. This is cosmetically a problem, especially if there is a difference between the two eyes. Even a 2- or 3-mm difference is noticeable. The normal aperture is 11 or 12 mm. If the upper lid covers the pupil, or as much as half the pupil, then vision may be affected. The ptosis may vary, and become worse when a person is tired. It may be congenital, hereditary, or acquired secondary to injury or a neurological problem. Testing of the visual field may show limitation of the upper half of vision, and therefore suggest that the indication for surgery is more than cosmetic. Surgical correction is complicated by the need of not only lifting the upper lid and trying to match it to the other eyelid, but doing so in such a way as to result in continued ability of the eyelid to blink and close normally, to protect the cornea. This procedure is best performed by an ophthalmic plastic surgeon, rather than a regular plastic surgeon.

Dermatochalasis

Dermatochalasis (commonly called, though incorrectly, blepharochalasis) is the term for the baggy drooping of stretched skin, usually of the upper eyelids. It is extremely common with increasing age, and often associated with being overweight, though it can occur in slender people, and can be hereditary. The degree varies from a mild cosmetic problem, to the point where the skin of the upper lid droops so much that vision is limited in the upper field of vision. Once the skin begins to stretch, it is advisable to avoid the temptation to rub the eyes, which can make it worse. Removal of the excess skin can be done, with good cosmetic and functional result. However, insurance and Medicare may not cover the expense of surgery if it seems to be only for cosmetic purposes.

Blepharospasm

This condition is not common and amounts to uncontrollable tendency for the eyelids to close involuntarily, transiently, or for increasing periods of time, varying from increased blinking to closure of the lids, with prolonged inability to open them to allow vision safely for, say, driving a car. Usually this is an idiopathic primary condition, but it can be a part of neurologic conditions such as Parkinsonism or Meige's Syndrome. Injection of botulinum toxin (Botox), into the facial nerve can show improvement for variable lengths of time, often months. This was one of the original uses of Botox, before "wrinkles."

Myokymia

This is a condition that involves involuntary twitching of the eyelids, upper or lower, or both. Sensation can vary from a feeling of fullness, to a twitching feeling, to being able to see the lid twitch in the mirror. Episodes are transient, brief, and variable in frequency. The usual expectation is for spontaneous cessation, though there may be occasional recurrence. Twitching is felt to be akin to nervousness, so a person becomes self-conscious and seeks ways to calm down. However, avoiding coffee, sleeping longer, or taking tranquilizers does not help. A person gets better anyway, and may as well perform as normally.

Lid Retraction

This is a situation whereby the upper lid actually pulls upward, making the eye or eyes appear larger. A small degree of this may be within normal limits, but a greater amount, especially if more in one eye than the other, may indicate thyroid hyperactive disease, and also especially if noted while looking downward. Worsening of the thyroid condition may also result in double vision, especially while looking upward, and bulging forward of the eye or eyes, called exophthalmos.

ITCHY EYES

Itchy Eyelids

These can be an acute or chronic problem. Acute problems include the hivelike reaction to something usually of foreign protein, such as an insect bite. Localized swelling can be remarkable, unaccompanied by redness or discharge, but of course associated with itching. This should be short-lived, and would be speeded in recovery by topical steroids or oral antihistamine. Chronic itching and redness, often accompanied by dry scaly dermatitis with wrinkling, is usually due to a contact dermatitis. This means the patient is handling something to which they are allergic, and spreading the allergy-causing material to the face by the hands. It is not necessary that the allergen be directly applied to the eye area. In a right-handed person, the right eye area is more likely to be involved. The skin around the eyes will be the first sign of this contact dermatitis, and a more generalized form eventually shows involvement of inside the elbows or underarms. Treatment involves recognizing the allergen, which may be something as common as a detergent or clothing dye, and avoiding contact with it. Topical steroid lotions relieve symptoms, but do not avoid recurrence. The most common medication causing such symptoms of allergy is Neomycin, which is contained in Neosporin and other antibiotic topical medications.

Itchy Eyeballs

These can be a significant problem and not so easy to diagnose as to the cause, but usually due to allergy. Symptoms can be a part of allergies such as hay fever, or as obvious as visiting a house with a cat present. The eyes become red and tearing. Relief can be obtained with a number of medications, but usually topical eye drops are better than oral anti-allergy medications.

There can be papillary changes in the conjunctiva, which are recognizable by a slit lamp (microscopic) exam, to help differentiate allergy from other causes of red eye, such as conjunctivitis. These can be so severe as to cause "giant papillae," most commonly seen with allergy to protein buildup on soft contact lenses. Before the introduction of daily wear disposable lenses, such allergic reaction often doomed a patient to not being able to wear soft contact lenses; but since disposable contact lenses, this giant papillary conjunctivitis type of allergy is rare.

Eye drops giving relief can be of the vasoconstrictor type, such as Visine or Vasocon, which are available without prescription. These medications give prompt, but temporary, relief. The unfortunate tendency to repeat use, at what can become shorter and shorter intervals, can result in rebound redness because of reflex vasodilatation, and actually make the eyes worse. So if it is desirable to take the red out for a special occasion, such as getting your picture taken, it is OK to use vasoconstrictor "take the red out" eye drops. However, if long-term relief is desired, prescription medications are available.

Prescription eye drops can be antihistamine, mast cell stabilizer, or anti-inflammatory in action, or a combination of these actions. Such medications may not be quite so rapid in relief effect, but can be continued for long-term effect during the allergy season. Steroid eye drops are among the best for prompt and lasting relief, but of course carry the possibility of long-term complications such as glaucoma (in a significant percentage of people) or cataracts (if used for a long time). NSAID (non steroidal anti-inflammatory drug (NSAID) eye drops are also available, which have similar, if not as reliable, effects as steroid drops, without the potential side effects. Less potent steroid drops have also been provided, which may give the positive beneficial effects of steroid drops, with greatly diminished chances of complications.

7

STRABISMUS (CROSS-EYED AND WALL-EYED)

Strabismus (strah-bis-mus) is a fancy term for the fact that the eyes are not straight. Most such problems are "primary," meaning origin from childhood development. Secondary strabismus may result from injury, neurologic, or medical problems.

Esotropia, being cross-eyed, may be from birth (congenital) or acquired. Being cross-eyed means that one eye is not straight; it is deviated internally toward the nose. If a child shows that the same eye is always crossed, then that eye is in danger of being amblyopic, and not developing normal vision. Some cross-eyed children can alternate freely, meaning that they can switch eyes, and use either eye quite well. These children are not at risk of amblyopia, but of course need professional reassurance about this. This is the goal of patching when treating amblyopia, to make the child see well with each eye. But, if the child can alternate fixation naturally, then patching may not be necessary to improve vision. However, patching may be used before surgery even if the vision seems equally good in each eye. This would be done to break up habits of suppression (ignoring one eye to avoid double vision), and get, perhaps, a binocular result from surgery.

The straightness of the eyes may be difficult to evaluate in early infancy, when the eyes may seem to drift once in a while. The vision and eye coordination takes time to develop. However, if it is apparent that a baby's eyes are really crossed, then the child should be examined even in early infancy. So if the baby's eyes still look crossed, only sometimes at age six months, this child should also be examined. A child age three can usually be taught the illiterate "E" game, and later expected to be able to know their "letters," so as to be able to read the "Snellen" chart. The frequency of preschool attendance these days has meant that more children are advanced in being able to read the ABC charts. This is good, because the results of reading a row of letters as in the Snellen ABC charts is more accurate than the illiterate E chart in reassuring that both eyes see equally well.

The goals of treatment of the cross-eyed child are basically three. The first, and most important, goal is to provide two eyes that see well, with or without glasses, even if they are not straight. The second goal is cosmetic, meaning that even if the eyes are not perfectly straight, they look straight. The third goal, and the most difficult to achieve, is that not only are the eyes looking straight, but they are straight—they both see well, and are working together binocularly (with stereopsis depth perception). To accomplish these goals may require patching, eye drops, glasses, surgery, or a combination of all these things. If the ultimate goal of binocular vision is obtained, then continued good result is expected. However, if fusion, or binocular result, is not obtained, then there is nothing to hold the eyes straight, so that an early good cosmetic surgical result may not last, and further surgery may be needed later.

The onset of becoming cross-eyed around age three is quite common, and is usually related to the need for glasses to correct farsightedness. This is because, at about this age, an accommodative-convergence relationship is developing, along with other coordination. This means that for each unit of accommodation, focusing to see up close, an expected demand for convergence is developed. Convergence means that the two eyes that are parallel for distance must move inward together so as to be looking at an object closer. The emmetropic eye, in perfect focus for distance, requires 3 diopters of focusing at 1/3 meter. Assuming both eyes are about the same, this normal relationship develops. Along with this focusing demand, there is also a "demand" for convergence of the eyes, so that they both point at an object 1/3 meter away. The "normal" reflex would mean that for every diopter of focusing, the eyes learn to converge an appropriate amount. Thus, for a close up distance of 1 meter, then 1 diopter of focusing is required, and the eyes must move inward to be converged to a distance of 1 meter.

Assuming that a child may be 3 diopters farsighted, then that child must focus or accommodate 3 diopters for distance, and another 3 diopters, or 6 diopters total, at 1/3 meter, twice the normal demand. This means that the child, in order to remain binocular, while focusing extra for distance, must ignore the excessive reflex demand to also converge at distance. Then, for close vision, this same child would have to reduce the amount of convergence being reflexively called for by more than the normal amount of focusing for this close distance. Using such an example, it is easy to understand how a child may become cross-eyed if very farsighted, because wearing glasses for 3 diopters of farsightedness means no stimulus to converge for distance, and no stimulus for extra convergence at 1/3 meter. Maintaining binocular vision without glasses is difficult under these circumstances, but children seem to do it in most cases, since the incidence of being cross-eyed is not equal to the amount of children who are farsighted to significant degree. So there must be other factors involved, including heredity.

The stimulus to overconverge results in crossing of the eyes, one eye fixating, and the other overconverged, or crossed. This type of acquired esotropia, related to being farsighted, is called accommodative esotropia. The eyes are usually straighter for distance and crossed more at near, for close work. The child is not expected to complain, as the brain is still adaptable. The brain avoids confusion by "suppressing" the image in the deviated eye. The child does not even know what is meant by "double vision." If not treated, amblyopia may result, just like in the child born cross-eyed.

The treatment, and possible cure, of accommodative esotropia is glasses, though it may become more complicated. As one may be able to understand, putting glasses on the 3-diopter farsighted child eliminates the demand for focusing at a distance, and reduces the accommodative demand for extra focusing at near, allowing the eyes to work together in more normal reflex action. However, once the eyes begin to cross, more than the basic glasses may be required. There seems to be an extra problem of overconvergence in many children, so that even with glasses that straighten the eyes for distance, there may be still a tendency to cross the eyes for close vision. Bifocals may correct this tendency, and sometimes eye drops can help. The goal, as usual, is to get the eyes working together in a binocular way, whatever it takes. Surgery may also be required. If binocular result can be obtained, then the child may go through life retaining this benefit. Since this extra "spastic" type reflex to overconverge at near reduces with maturation, the need for glasses will change. The bifocals will probably not be required as the child matures, and even the need for glasses may be reduced to a part-time need. Contact lenses may become an option. Reportedly, a Heisman trophy winner, the quarterback on the USC No. 1 football team in the nation, has gone through these steps, bifocal glasses, and surgery, and apparently has achieved binocular results. This may be among his greatest accomplishments.

Surgery for esotropia (cross-eyes) can be quite successful, but success must be tempered by overall result. The goals must be considered preoperatively. If both eyes see well, other treatments have been utilized to achieve this status, and a binocular result is the goal, then it must be understood that glasses and other treatments may be necessary to maintain a good result postoperatively. These muscles are normally quite strong, able to do perhaps 100 times the power required, but expected to work in a delicate coordination with other muscles. Surgery may then be compared to doing an orthopedic type procedure for a neurologic problem, or more crudely, a carpentry management for an electronic problem. Treatment of the neurologic (electronic) portion, of course, refers to need for glasses, patching, and so forth. The amount of surgery is determined by the amount of crossing of the eyes, *with corrective glasses*, not the amount of crossing without glasses. This is difficult for parents to understand. As mentioned, if glasses are needed postoperatively, they eventually may not be needed once a good result has been maintained neurologically, a binocular result. If the amount of surgery is performed to make the eyes straight without glasses, then the farsighted child is too likely to become exotropic (walleyed) later in life, an overcorrection. Exercises, though well designed, are not as effective as glasses, bifocals, eye drops, or surgery in correcting esotropia and amblyopia.

The example of becoming cross-eyed around age three as indication of accommodative type acquired esotropia is illustrative, and basically true, but there seem to be other factors, often hereditary. For example, probably the majority of farsighted children, 3 diopters more or less, do not become cross-eyed and seem to accomplish normal binocularity. In regard to hereditary factors, I recollect a lovely young lady who brought her third son, her third child, in for exam. She was fully expecting that the fact that since she herself had been cross-eyed, needing glasses and eventually contact lenses to keep her eyes straight, and since her first two sons had followed in her path (both observed in the back of the room wearing their glasses), that this youngest son was also destined the same fate. When I told her that this son was not cross-eyed and was not expected to need glasses, a faint smile crossed her face. I interpreted this to mean that it may be worth another try for a girl, and maybe one who would not be cross-eyed.

Pseudostrabismus can result from a condition called epicanthus, a fold in the skin toward the nose that is quite common in Asians, but occurs in all races. Children with this condition can appear to be cross-eyed, even when the eyes are perfectly straight. Whenever the child looks slightly left of right, the skin covers part of the eye making it look crossed. Then when the child's nose grows, the skin is pulled away from the eye, and the child no longer looks cross-eyed, which results in the impression that the child "out grew" being cross-eyed. I recall examining a small child of Scandinavian extraction years ago. His mother had reassured me that her child was cross-eyed, but would outgrow the problem like his older siblings. Since they were nearby, I invited the other siblings of this large family into the room. They demonstrated stages of nose growth and diminishing degree of epicanthus, confirming that none of them had ever been cross-eyed. However, such a story of "outgrowing" being cross-eyes is a bad influence on parents who delay bringing their children in for treatment.

Exotropia, the outward turning of one, eye is a different problem in many ways. The onset is usually later, so that early onset in infancy can signal other neurological problem. There are other differences. Contrary to esotropic children, amblyopia is not expected with exotropia. In addition, a form of binocular vision is usually maintained, accompanied by a type of situational suppression to avoid double vision. In other words, the child may have normal depth perception much of the time, but when one eye drifts outward, the vision is selectively suppressed in that eye so as to not be annoyed by diplopia (double vision). The apparent onset of exotropia may not be evident until adult life, but the lack of diplopia is a factor, meaning that the actual onset was in early childhood. Usually one eye drifts when looking at a distance, intermittently at first, but the condition may progress to the point where one eye is turned outward all the time, even for close vision.

In the meantime, the exotropic patient does not complain. Parents and others may notice drifting out of one eye, and since it seems intermittent, and controlled by blinking or parents yelling instructions to straighten the eye, parents sometimes think they are responsible to control the child's eyes, by constant reminder. One symptom is the apparent light sensitivity of the exotropic patient outdoors. First of all, the tendency for one eye to drift is usually for distance, as outdoors in sunlight, and usually signified by closing one eye. The patient is unaware of this, since he or she is not unaware of double vision, and unaware that the closure of one eye outdoors is actually to avoid a form of double vision, which apparently cannot be so easily ignored in sunlight. Such people are not truly photosensitive, or they would have to close or squint both eyes. If the outward turning becomes worse, the patients feels that people are not looking at them in conversation, because of the natural tendency of people to look at the wrong eye, the outward-turned, eye. This makes a patient feel uncomfortable. Also, other people may think that exotropic patients have a shifty or untrustworthy appearance, since they do not appear to look others in the eye.

Treatment of exotropia may involve glasses, if the patient is nearsighted, since the glasses would have straightening effect, but surgery may become necessary if the problem becomes severe. There is not the urgency involved as with esotropia, since amblyopia is not expected. Also, the problem does not always get worse and may even spontaneously get better. Surgical correction can be quite successful, but cannot be guaranteed to be permanent. Actually, it is all right to consider cosmetic goals as an indicator. In other words, if the problem is barely noticeable, then there is less indication for surgery. Another factor, however, is that insurance is more likely to cover the surgery in childhood than adult life, when the procedure may be considered cosmetic by the insurance company. Postoperatively, double vision can be temporarily expected, and this is not all bad, since a more permanent result may then be expected when the double vision goes away.

Secondary strabismus refers to situations where the eyes that were once binocular, or working together, lose binocularity. This, of course, results in double vision (diplopia). This is also in contrast to the person in childhood who develops misalignment of the eyes and, if young enough, can ignore one eye so as to avoid double vision. Causes of secondary strabismus can vary from injury, to surgery, disease such as thyroid problem, neurologic disease such as stroke or multiple sclerosis, or not uncommonly, cause unknown. Once binocularity has been accomplished, the eyes have some degree of ability to keep themselves straight, a kind of fine-tuning, which can be compared to the fine-tuning of a TV set. The outward-turning tendency can be overcome by convergence, a very powerful ability of most people in order to avoid double vision, like a horizontal hold adjustment of a TV. The ability to overcome the crossing tendency is less, and requires divergence, the outward-turning ability of the eyes. The vertical separation of images is the most difficult for the eyes to overcome, and usually requires a prism in the glasses to avoid double vision. Of these fine-tuning abilities, the only one practically treated by exercises is convergence. So the primary indication for eye exercises is for convergence insufficiency, especially demonstrated in reading problems. This is either primarily a problem, such as in nearsighted people, especially if they do not wear their glasses for reading, or a secondary one, such as in head injuries. Of interest is the fact that the greatest disability is in cases where the images are close together, but separated. This type diplopia is very annoying and confusing. When the images are far apart, it is easier to ignore one image, and concentrate on the other. In cases where the images are close together, a little prism in the glasses may help a lot by bringing the images together. However, if the double vision varies, as when looking right or left, then prisms will not work.

If the eyes were binocular before diplopia (double vision) occurred, then there is a good chance that the two eyes will regain fusion, the use of the eyes together, once there is improvement in the problem that caused the secondary strabismus, such as in stroke recovery. In the meantime, it is important to encourage binocular use of the eyes, such as allowing head turn or tilt to avoid diplopia, rather than cover one eye. Covering one eye is a temporary relief of diplopia, but may delay spontaneous recovery. Exercises, if utilized, may be given false credit for spontaneous neurological improvement, since the problem is usually not weak muscles, but temporary lack of neurological input.

Secondary strabismus may also result from loss of vision in one eye. The so-called fusion-free position of a blind eye is to be crossed in childhood, and to be outward turned or exotropic in adult life. Such may be the expectations for a blind eye from injury. An eye crossed in childhood for such reason may however seem to straighten with age, but eventually turn outward in adult life. Such can also be the case for an amblyopic eye, going from being crossed in childhood to exotropic later in life, even if there has been no surgery.

PART III

AGE-RELATED EYE PROBLEMS (GETTING OLD AIN'T FOR SISSIES)

8

PRESBYOPIA

The treatment of age-related hearing disorder, called presbycusis, is amplification. The treatment of age-related vision loss, called presbyopia, is magnification. Presbycusis is quite likely. Presbyopia is predictably inevitable.

The eye, having gone through normal development, reaches full size, and has great powers of accommodation, or focusing. Eventually about 10 diopters or units of focusing ability develop, and are retained through the twenties's in age. The accommodation gradually reduces in our thirties, until it begins to be a noticeable problem in focusing up close by mid forties, at which time it has dropped to 3 diopters, giving a near point of about twelve inches. So when one has had a few "Jack Benny Birthdays" (he was thirty-nine when he died), reading help is needed, even if vision was "perfect" before. The arms get "too short," because the closer small objects are brought to the eyes (not just for reading, but any small object), the more the focusing limitation is evident. Good light, like standing by a lamp, or window, or using a flashlight can help, at least temporarily.

Presbyopia is an age-related problem, but not believed to be due to old or weak focusing muscles. Thoughts along these lines have suggested eye exercises or special diets, but such experiments are not fruitful, other than psychologically. The acceptable theory, is that decrease of accommodation due to age, is due to sclerosis, or hardening of the lens of the eye, such that focusing muscular effort gets less result. One of the problems in evaluating age-related focusing problems, is that most estimates are based on subjective factors, which involve too many variables, such as lighting, amount of rest, and so forth. A basic factor not considered by most people, is that any distance problem need be considered or corrected before one can adequately evaluate the close-up or reading problems. In other words, if the distance vision is not perfect, and can be corrected by glasses for myopia, astigmatism, or hyperopia, then the close-up vision is affected, more than just the age-related expectations. This brings up the subject of glasses, the usual treatment of presbyopia. The reading problem is added to any existing distance imperfection. The nearsighted person, wearing their glasses, experiences trouble reading also, and needs something different for reading than they do for distance. Same for the farsighted or astigmatic person. For most of us, who are emmetropic, there was no previous problem, and the eyes may continue to see quite well for distance without glasses. This makes the need for glasses, for the first time, perhaps even more surprising. The emmetropic situation exists in about forty per cent of the population, and therefore the largest group.

There are *three* kinds of reading glasses. What most people think of as reading glasses are what are called single-vision reading glasses. This means that the whole full sized lens is the reading correction, in a full sized frame. Actually, eventually, this becomes the worst of the three choices for reading glasses due to lack of versatility. A person has to slide the glasses down, and look over them to see TV or distance objects. Those who choose such reading glasses may do so for different reasons, such as emphasizing that they are almost perfect, but sometimes need reading glasses.

Those who wish to wear glasses at a minimum can accomplish this goal with single-vision reading glasses, because it is too inconvenient to wear them much. As time goes on, stronger reading glasses will be required to see small objects, causing more and more of a shut-in feeling when looking across the room. In practice, I have experienced rare reasons whereby single-vision reading glasses are justifiably best. In one instance, a steel worker working on skyscrapers said that it was required as a welder, that he have single-vision close-up glasses, so that he would not even consider taking a step away from his work with his reading glasses on. Another man, a Union negotiator, described how he successfully controlled negotiations by putting on his glasses to read contracts, then removing them to respond, then slowly repeating this process, to give him time to think and stall the opposition. Probably the most common reason for getting single-vision reading glasses is that a person can try them on in the drug store, and if they seem to help, think that they can avoid an eye examination. Another stated and practical reason is that they are cheap, and a person keeps losing them, because they have to take them off to do something else.

A second type of reading glasses are called Half Eyes. These are smaller glasses that fit lower, commonly called Ben Franklins (who strangely enough actually is credited with inventing the bifocal). With half-eyes, someone with good distance vision can look over the glasses easily to see at a distance. Another advantage, is that such glasses may be worn higher for computer use. In my experience, people either love half eyes or hate them, with little attitude in between. Among the disadvantages include that they usually do not fit well, and tend to slide down. When I see people walking around wearing their half-eyes, too busy to take them off, then I conclude that they are ready for the third kind of reading glasses, the bifocal. The main complications of starting out with over-the-counter reading glasses are: (1) People think they have solved their eye problem and do not need an eye exam, even though the age of discovery of reading problems is also the age when age-related eye diseases may appear. (2) Starting with such glasses frequently makes it difficult to adjust to multifocals, especially to the no line bifocal called the progressive lens.

The mention of the word bifocal can result in significant reaction in people, and commonly negative. Many believe that the word bifocal means need to wear glasses constantly, and most feel they neither need or desire to wear glasses full time. Actually, a bifocal is just one of three choices of reading glasses, and full time wear is not required. It just provides more versatility in the long run, and along with half-eyes are the better choices for the emmetropic person, one who continues to have good distance vision, as to initial reading glasses. If a person likes to wear sunglasses, they need to understand that eventually the bifocal will be needed in the sunglasses. However, after going through the whole discussion as to the pros and cons of the *three* types of reading glasses with the presbyope getting their first reading glasses, the usual response is, "I just want the reading glasses." This means, of course, that they have not listened or preferred not to listen to my presentation. Hey, I am used to it. What they want, of course, is single-vision reading glasses. Want and need, of course, are sometimes different.

If there is any distance problem of potential significance, then the bifocal should be the easy choice, at least logically. However, logic does not always win out. Reasons offered against a bifocal include:

Question: Why do I need a bifocal if I only need reading glasses?
Answers:
1. Even if distance vision is perfect, it will become convenient to be able to leave the glasses on when busy, and requiring vision at all distances.
2. If safety glasses are required at work, they need to be a bifocal to allow vision safely at all distances, and yet cover the eye for protection.
3. If you like to wear sunglasses, you will eventually need a bifocal sun glass to be able to see small things up close, usually by age 50–60. If a golfer, the sports bifocal may involve a small bifocal segment placed low enough as to not get in the way for putting, but yet enough help in case you get a "small score."
4. If you work with computers, and need to see at all distances, then you will be eventually a candidate for a trifocal. However, one first must become accustomed to a bifocal, and then note that there is a problem for intermediate distances, as eventually noted somewhere in the 50–60 age range. Just as one needs to be able to walk before learning to run, one needs to become accustomed to a bifocal before learning to use trifocals. When this proper sequence is taken, most people say that the trifocals were easier to adjust to than their first bifocal, especially if well motivated, as in computer use. Actually, of course, trifocals are superior to bifocals, eventually as an upgrade. They are also, just an alternative for someone who wants to see everything at the appropriate age. A person does not have to go to a trifocal however, if satisfied with their bifocal. More will be said about trifocals later.

Question: If I am nearsighted, and can see up close satisfactorily by taking off my distance glasses, why do I need a bifocal?

Answer: You may be able to see well up close without glasses due to your nearsightedness, and this may continue to be true, depending on how nearsighted you are. However, by using a bifocal you have the choice of leaving the glasses on to see up close, or taking them off, if convenient. Here are some common situations:

1. Some have never worn their glasses to read, dating back to first glasses for nearsightedness, either by confusion or false information. Young people can focus quite well, and there are no health or practical reasons to remove the glasses for reading, especially in the classroom situation. Such myopes become prematurely presbyopic, meaning that they cannot read with their glasses on at earlier age, maybe in their thirties. Their eyes become "lazy" when it comes to focusing, since they can see without glasses with little or no focusing effort at near, and are not used to the normal amount of focusing required for close work with glasses on.

2. Though they once wore their glasses most of the time, and now that they are forced to remove them for close work, they end up not wearing their glasses so much, unless forced to, like for driving a car. Such people have traded routinely good distance vision, for a compromise based on need for close-up vision.

3. Those mildly or moderately nearsighted, have rather "in between" vision naturally, meaning that the distance vision is not terribly bad, and near vision is pretty good, to a degree, but it is eventually no longer as good as it should be. Such people may be difficult to convince to get a bifocal, and when given a choice may want two pair of glasses, one for distance, and one for near. This means three alternatives: No glasses, reading glasses, and distance glasses. No glasses will be the usual choice. However, if having a bifocal, there are now only two choices: No glasses or glasses that allow improvement of vision for both distance and near (and part-time wear is fine).

4. Along with desire to avoid bifocals, some wonder about the choice of going to contact lenses. Generally contact lenses are worn by nearsighted people, and to a lesser extent by farsighted people. Those waiting until the age of presbyopia, before starting contact lenses for nearsightedness, have waited too long and often make their situation worse. The alternative of removing their glasses for close work is no longer practical, and their need for glasses is switched from their original help for distance, to needing help for up close in the form of reading glasses. Myopes are better off to go to contact lenses prior to the presbyopic age. On the other hand, some farsighted people are quite happy to go into contact lenses in the presbyopic age. Many of these people have not accepted the fact that they have a distance problem, and remember well when they could see at all distances without glasses. Such people often adapt well to monovision contact lenses, meaning one eye sees better for distance, and the other for near. Monovision is also often quite successful as an alternative to the nearsighted person already wearing contact lenses when they become presbyopic. The emmetrope, one who still sees well at distance with both eyes, can wear one contact lens for close work, another type

of monovision. However, most people have trouble adjusting to just one contact lens, even if a soft contact lens.

5. Contact lenses wearers, of course become presbyopic too, making the wear of contact lenses less motivating, if the main reason is to avoid glasses. The contact lens wearer is advised that it is OK to use over-the-counter or drug store reading glasses, since the contact lenses usually make both eyes balanced in good distance vision, and such "drug store" glasses are for people whose eyes are equally in need for reading, and have no significant uncorrected astigmatism. Often, the nearsighted contact lens wearer, when becoming presbyopic, may be less motivated and switches back to wearing glasses. However, contact lens wearers have options, including the same as the emmetropic person, that is part-time reading help, including bifocals. Also, as mentioned, monovision fitting can be successful.

Bifocal contact lenses have been available for years with limited success, and are being advertised lately as if a new alternative. These multi focal lenses have some problems due to haloes and distortions, such that the average contact lens wearer would prefer the sharper vision obtained with their original contact lenses, and usually prefer to go to monovision as a preferable approach to solving reading problems.

6. Those who have worn glasses full time for most of their life, usually adjust rapidly to bifocals and trifocals. Some are so nearsighted that reading without glasses is not very practical, because of having to hold things too close. Others, with astigmatism, cannot see well at any distance without their glasses. Sometimes, however, those with significant astigmatism do not become aware of a problem until they have presbyopia added to their basic problem with astigmatism. Naturally, a bifocal is the best choice of reading glasses, so that they can also see what they have been missing for distance. However, adjustment may be difficult if they have not become used to wearing glasses, and much patience is required to get used to seeing things properly. Tilting and distortion of images can be expected by those whose astigmatism has been uncorrected, but such people need to be assured that this all will go away as they adjust to their glasses. Wearing a bifocal, in this situation, may be mainly for reading. There then is the expectation that eventually the distance portion will be appreciated at some point, and this will be a good sign. For example, many such people could not pass a drivers test without glasses, and if they have it put on their driver's license that glasses are required, they are in danger of being cited for not wearing their glasses if they have not allowed themselves to become adjusted.

Question: Why should I get a bifocal, when I feel I can still see good for distance, and I am farsighted? But reading is really becoming a problem now. I really did not feel I have a distance problem, until demonstrated in my eye exam, and I still don't quite believe it. Why can't I just have 2 pair of glasses, one part time for distance, and one part time for reading?

Answer: A bifocal will be the best choice for reading glasses. You would never get your money's worth out of a separate pair of distance glasses. They would not get worn, and you would never know where you left them. But if you get a bifocal, you can see what you are missing for distance, and then decide if you will wear them more than just for reading. The reading need would still be primary, and the distance need be secondary. It is expected that any distance improvement will be especially appreciated at night, as in driving a car. If you decide you need to wear the bifocal mainly for reading, that is all right. Then later, if you recognize some need or help for distance, you can wear them more, as you wish. If you have trouble wearing them for walking, then don't wear them for walking around. But also remember that the other choices of reading glasses are even worse for walking around, and that with a bifocal you have the potential of being able to leave them on more of the time.

Some people, since they are so certain they need nothing for distance, or because they think wearing a distance correction may make their eyes "weak," want nothing in the top of their bifocal. Such a person, if, 1 diopter farsighted, and old enough to need an extra 2 diopters for reading (age 50+), would have a big jump to go from nothing for distance, and all of sudden go to 3 diopters of help for near work. The jump from +1 diopter in the top, or distance portion, to another +2 diopters in the bottom of the bifocal, is easier to tolerate. Another example, using numbers, is a female patient of mine who had a bifocal previously prescribed, with nothing in the top, and +1.00 in the bottom. Our exam demonstrated that she was 1 diopter farsighted, and also needed another +1 reading addition, a total of +2 need for reading. She returned saying that she could not understand why she could no longer see better for distance, by throwing her head back so that she could see through the lower bifocal, for distance. When asked if she could see all right through the top part of the bifocal, and better for reading, she said "well, yes." So, in general, if a person thinks they would rather have 2 pair of glasses, one pair should be a bifocal.

There is another interesting phenomenon which enters into adjusting to glasses. The size of objects can seem to vary, depending on whether a person is in need for glasses for farsightedness or nearsightedness. To give an example, the emmetropic person can see the 20/20 line without glasses for distance. The nearsighted person needs glasses to see the 20/20 line, but it is an image actually smaller than that seen by the emmetrope. The farsighted person wearing glasses, sees the 20/20 line bigger than the emmetrope. The person wearing contact lenses has the magnification factor "normalized," such that the nearsighted and the farsighted have no magnification difference from the emmetropic person. The nearsighted person is often surprised to note that things look bigger with contact lenses on, compared to how seen with their glasses. The farsighted person, however, is one who does not get glasses so early, and often not until they become presbyopic. For them, with their first glasses, they not only have to get used to the impression that things seem a bit blurred for distance (though really not), but that things look bigger, and therefore closer. With contact lenses, the object size is more normalized, not as big as with spectacles.

Question: Why have my eyes become "weaker" since I started to wear glasses? I used to have excellent vision, and was a pilot in the air force. Since I started to wear glasses, in my forties, I now need bifocals all the time. My distance vision is bad also. I sometimes think that if I never started wearing glasses, I would not be so bad as I am now.

Answer: Your question and description of your dilemma are quite understandable. However, it is not the fault of your glasses that you now need to wear your bifocal full time. You are probably farsighted, not terribly, or you would not have been a pilot. But a young person can be one or two diopters farsighted, able to pass a flight physical, and not be aware any problem. However, when presbyopia adds need for another one or two diopters for reading, the latent farsightedness becomes evident. By then it is also difficult to focus the extra one or two diopters for distance. As discussed, it may take awhile to recognize the distance problem, but once adjusting to the glasses, it is logical that seeing without glasses seems much worse than it once was. It is not unusual for a farsighted person to select drug store reading glasses, only to discover that they gave not bad vision for distance, and they needed a higher number to see for reading. So the bifocal, or glasses in general, do not make the eyes weaker, as may be the common impression. And yes, it is normal for the farsighted person to note progressive need for the glasses to be worn.

The good news about this, is that a person does not have to look for their glasses so much, because they are wearing them. This is because a person tends to select good vision, with glasses, compared to poor vision, and not because the glasses have made their eyes "weaker." This is actually a better result than for the person who never tries the bifocal, throws the glasses aside and says that they never will be able to wear a bifocal. One of my senior patients, when asked why he did not wear a bifocal, stated that he was given a bifocal, went out and played golf with them, and never shot such a bad game of golf in his life, so he threw them away and vowed to never try again. Such a person's impatience may result a lifetime of not seeing well, and fussing with multiple pairs of glasses, which never seem right. Certainly, postponing the adjustment, like waiting "until I really need them" makes it even more difficult to adjust to what is really needed. And if you wait too long, then there may be no use "bugging" you, for as in the case of my patient with bad golf experience, it may become too late to try new things.

Choices of Bifocals, Trifocals, Etc.

The old fashioned bifocal had a round top and was cosmetically not bad, but the usefulness was limited by design, and is now prescribed mainly to elderly people who are accustomed to only this style of bifocal.

The standard bifocal has a straight-line top, to separate distance vision from near vision, with appropriate help. The line may go part way or completely across the lens, as in an "executive" bifocal. The executive bifocal is good, but the top line is quite prominent, and looking side to side does not require a bifocal segment all across the lens for near work. One needs to get used to the "line" at first, but awareness of the "line" just seems to go away with time. And, if compared to half-eye reading glasses, this line is no different than the top frame of the half-eyes.

The no-line bifocal, called the progressive bifocal, cosmetically looks just like single-vision glasses, no different from glasses worn prior to presbyopia, or from single-vision reading glasses. There is a graduated change from distance correction to full near correction, such that features of a "trifocal" are present, from the beginning. This type reading glasses has cosmetic appeal, and is quite useful, but has a small reading area compared to other choices, big enough, but smaller than what one may have become used to, such as half-eyes or single-vision readers.

There are expected problems of adjustment to first bifocals, with or without the line. If one has become used to other kinds of reading glasses, like half-eyes, or single-vision reading glasses, then certain problems may be predictable, since the reading area of these original glasses is quite larger. Such people probably would adjust easier to the standard bifocal, with a line, since the reading area is larger than the reading area in the progressive reading add. There are also some distortions with the progressive add initially, which are temporary. If, however, the progressive add is your first pair of reading glasses, or if you are a person accustomed to wearing glasses full time for distance, and now needs additional help for reading, the progressive add may be as easy to adjust to as the bifocal with the line, or easier. Another advantage of progressive add multifocals, is that once one is accustomed to them, then getting used to stronger glasses is easier than with a standard bifocal, and there is no need to go to a "trifocal."

Then what is a trifocal, and why would that be needed? When a person has reached the fifties in age, they usually need 2 diopters reading addition. When this happens, if not before, such people note that there is an area, in between, that is not covered by the bifocal—typically arm's length away. This is especially noted now that so many people are using computers, which are further away in working distance than usual reading distance. The person with a bifocal notes that they have to tip their chin up to look through the bifocal, and move forward to get into focus. This is awkward, inconvenient, and sometimes uncomfortable. With a trifocal, a person does not need to raise the chin so high, and one does not need to move forward, because things are in focus at arms length distance. People with trifocals also may be noticed to be looking through the trifocal intermediate segment in the conversation distance. One potential disadvantage is the notation that your friends may have wrinkles.

It is natural to assume that trifocals would be difficult for adjustment, but if a person starts with a standard bifocal, and wants to see everything, and is as well motivated as computer users, the usual response is that the trifocal was not as difficult as the first bifocal. Like the bifocal, the higher line becomes not noticeable eventually, as one gets used to the glasses. Some trifocal wearers wear just bifocals in their sunglasses, but others want the trifocal in all glasses. By the way, I have had patients who came back with a progressive lens, thinking that this is a "trifocal." Actually, the progressive lens has "features" of a trifocal, but is not a true trifocal. The person who has had a standard bifocal would be expected to adjust better to the standard trifocal, with two lines, rather than the progressive add.

Those who have had an executive bifocal, one that has a line going all the way across the lens, may also want an executive trifocal. This can be done, but a more practical trifocal is what is called and ED trifocal. This trifocal has an intermediate segment line that goes all the way across the lens, but the bifocal segment is more of a regular segment bifocal, with a line that does not go all the way across. The reason for this, is that it is more common to scan side to side while doing computer or other intermediate distance work than it is in reading. Also, two lines going all the way across can be more confusing when looking around in a scanning situation, like railroad tracks.

Once, after discussing trifocals with a lady working in an office with computers, I was given an important reason for denial. She said, "I agree, from what you have said, that I need a trifocal, but I am not going to get trifocals. You see there are a lot of girls in the office, all about the same age, and I am not going to be the first one in trifocals."

CONTACT LENSES AS AN ALTERNATIVE IN PRESBYOPIA

Contact lenses are not the best alternative for management of presbyopia. There are such things as bifocal contact lenses and multi focal lenses, but they are not very successful. Problems include seeing halos around lights and reduced contrast sensitivity, blurred vision. More success has been obtained, in those already wearing contact lenses, by going to what is called monovision. That means keeping one eye, usually the right eye in a right handed person, seeing well for distance, and using the other eye for seeing at near. If there is not too great a difference between the two eyes, this can work quite well, at least for a while.

Most contact lens wearers are nearsighted. They begin wearing contact lenses, usually at a young age, and they then become like an emmetropic person, one who sees well at any distance without glasses, until they become presbyopic, by age forty to forty-five. At this age, then the contact lens wearer can begin wearing reading glasses, part time, and have the choice of any of the three kinds of reading glasses available. Also, since the contact lenses balance the eyes for distance, any of the reading glasses available "over the counter" will work, or what I call "drug store glasses," at least at first, when they are convincing themselves that they really need them. And though these people once wore prescription glasses of quality, it is interesting that they may continue wearing unattractive ill-fitting drug store glasses, as if to emphasize that they really don't need glasses, or at least, not much.

Though most contact lens wearers are nearsighted, farsighted contact lens wearers are often among the happiest with monovision. The hyperopic, or farsighted, person usually saw quite well without glasses until adult life, usually prematurely noting reading problems, before the usual presbyopic age. At first, the problem seems mainly for reading, then distance becomes a problem also, and monovision makes them more happy. They often feel as if seeing like they did before they needed glasses. Emmetropic people can do monovision also, but this usually means wearing only one soft contact lens, for the reading eye. It can be done, but actually there are few who have the motivation to master this approach to management of presbyopia. By the way, monovision contact lens wear requires that both eyes see well. If one drops down in vision, for example due to a cataract, then it becomes a problem as to which way to use the second best eye, for distance or for close work.

Monovision is actually a compromise. Two eyes are better than one. Therefore, vision with bifocal glasses is better, but, as mentioned, this is not often successful with contact lens bifocals. Monovision is quite successful until about the mid-fifties in age. When the needed reading power of the "reading eye" is greater than +1.50 or +1.75, binocular vision is threatened. The reading requirements of someone age 50 or greater, increases from +1.75 to +2.00, and gradually up to +2.50 (full strength). If an attempt is made to make the reading eye "keep up" with these needs, the patient begins to feel uncomfortable, and if they can express the problem, like using one eye at a time. They have lost binocularity, though they may actually be able to read better with the stronger reading contact lens. I have seen some people, however, who though they have lost their binocularity, see well for reading, and are not complaining, so are allowed to continue wearing the stronger lens for reading. The motor vehicle department does not like, or understand monovision, but usually is unaware of the situation.

It is probably better to accept the "compromise" situation with monovision, by leaving the "reading eye" at only +1.50 or +1.75. With this, people are usually satisfied in most situations, even into more senior age. Only sometimes is there a need to see better. People may say that, sometimes they feel like a need to remove the contact lenses and put on the distance glasses when driving, especially at night. Other times, it is noted that for prolonged reading, a person may feel that it is better to remove the contact lenses, and either wear glasses, or read without glasses, if suitably nearsighted. For solving the reading problem, monovision contact lens wearers, rather than removing their contact lenses, may revert to the drug store reading glasses. Such glasses are obviously wrong, since they treat both eyes the same, and with monovision, one eye needs less help than the other. The best solution is, guess what, a bifocal to wear over the contact lenses.

A natural response to this suggestion, is that the reason a person is wearing contact lenses is to avoid glasses, like bifocals. A lot of the resistance is again based on the idea that bifocals are for full time glasses wear. On the contrary, in this circumstance especially, the bifocal is meant to be only part time, and as a way to assure more full time contact lens wear. The bifocal would be put on when driving at night, or for distance vision, to use the top part, which bring the reading eye up to good distance vision, and of course have nothing in the top for the distance seeing eye, or maybe a bit for uncorrected astigmatism. Driving home at night, or to a party, then means popping on the bifocal so as to see well for driving. When destination arrived, the glasses are removed and usual vision with contact lenses enjoyed. Then, when needing to read better, the bifocals also could be popped on temporarily, until not needing to see so perfectly, which would be expected to be most of the time. The bifocals would be a better choice than drug store glasses for reading, and no glasses for distance, or a separate pair of distance glasses which would not be worn, because then one cannot see well up close. Most of the time, probably 95 percent of the time, the bifocals would not be needed, and the monovision contact lens wearer would continue to function well without glasses.

9

CATARACTS

Other than presbyopia, the most common age-related eye problem is cataract.

Cataracts are also inevitable. You will hear things suggesting wearing sunglasses or taking nutrients to avoid cataract, but, if we live long enough, we all get cataracts. It can be said that the same process that makes the lens more rigid with age, results first in presbyopia, and then, in advanced form, causes in cataracts. Sixty percent of our population over the age of sixty have cataracts, and 70 percent of those over age seventy-five have cataracts. Cataract means clouding of the lens of the eye. There are different kinds, but all progressively block out light, which has passed through the pupil, from reaching the retina, in the back of the eye. The camera comparison is that the pictures turn out dimmer, and less colorful. Most cataracts are very slow in development, especially the most common, those age-related. Secondary cataracts may occur from use of steroids, trauma, or diabetes, and these may be more rapid in development. Congenital cataracts are rare, fortunately, since visual results are often not so good after treatment. In most cases, if vision has had a chance to develop normally, and there is nothing else wrong with the eye, then the vision is usually well restored after cataract removal.

Hereditary cataracts occur, but are not common. If family history describes cataracts in relatives in their seventies or eighties, or above, then this probably just suggests long familial life spans and age-related cataracts. Cataracts occurring in younger people, in their forties or fifties, may suggest a hereditary tendency.

So a cataract is any opacity of the lens of the eye. Depending on how much this opacity blocks the pupil, the vision is progressively blurred. When the vision is bad enough, then cataract surgery may be performed. This, of course, depends on the subjective desire to see better. Many people are not even aware of their vision change until it is pointed out to them in the course of an eye examination. Some are so worried about their cataracts that they have to be reassured that we are not dealing with something like a cancer that has to be treated early. Age is another concern, but we can assure that there is no such thing as being too old, or almost too sick, to have cataract surgery. It is done under local anesthesia, and as an outpatient procedure. It is also true that many people never get enough effect on their vision that they need to have their cataracts removed before they are deceased.

The change in vision from cataracts is usually quite slow, especially in what is called "cortical cataracts." Cortical cataracts are like spokes of clouded areas starting in the periphery of the lens, and working centrally. Another kind of cataract, posterior subcapsular cataract, is an opacity as if painted centrally on the back surface of the lens. This kind of cataract may progress more rapidly, and can be hereditary, due to diabetes, or result from use of oral steroids, such as prednisone. A third type of cataract, nuclear sclerosis, is also usually slow in development. However, it can cause nuisance by "myopic shift." This means that the eye may become more nearsighted than it was, or if farsighted, less farsighted, so that glasses may need changing more frequently than normal, to keep up with distance vision needs. Such cataracts are responsible for the "tale of second sight." A fella says, "I used to have eyes like an eagle and could shoot a squirrel off a tree limb a block away. Then my arms got too short, and I needed reading glasses. The other day, I noticed that I can read without glasses again; I have got 'Second Sight.'" His friend inquires, "How about squirrel hunting?" Fella says, "Nope, can't see across the street so well anymore." Such a story suggests the diagnosis of cataract, without need for examination.

The usual criterion as to whether a cataract is ready for surgery has to do with being able to pass a DMV or driver's license visual test, usually requiring 20/40 vision (in California). Actually, only one eye is required to pass a driver's test, but it is also logical that some sort of explanation be provided as to why the other eye does not see well enough to pass the vision test. Often, the reason is that a person should be wearing corrective glasses, so failure to pass a driver's test may trigger a need for your eye doctor to complete a vision evaluation form in order to get a driver's license. Anyway, if vision has failed in the cataract patient to the point that one eye does not see well enough to pass the driver's vision test, then this person has waited long enough, and now generally qualifies for cataract surgery, even if one does not drive a car. Of course, this is not a rigid criterion, and certainly a person does not have to undergo surgery if he or she does not want to see better. However, it is also true, that to postpone surgery because of fear of the procedure is not justified, if one can become familiar with the details of surgery, local anesthesia, and the minimal postoperative limitations.

The 20/40 guideline for establishing the need for cataract surgery is a standard conservative approach to recommending cataract surgery. Actually, the patient determines when it is time, because of the need to see better. Some patients need a pep talk to get them ready to decide to have surgery, and others are almost too eager. As mentioned, some patients think the cataract needs to be gotten out of there, like some sort of cancer. It is also true that some people may be able to see as well as 20/25 or 20/30, but be bothered by glare at night. When exposed to a bright light, such as headlights from an oncoming car, their vision can be shown to drop to more dangerous levels for driving. The patient and surgeon may then agree something needs to be done. Amazingly you may hear ads for eye drops, specifically Similisan, as useful to "relieve symptoms of cataracts," and emphasizing that there are no harmful side effects. Since the symptoms of cataract involve blurred vision to a variable degree, any success of such drops would be expected to be psychological and the lack of side effects due to the inactivity of the ingredients. Readers, having learned about cataracts, should not be confused by such claims.

What about waiting for a cataract to get "ripe," a term you may have heard. Well, this is a rather "old-fashioned" concept that needs explaining. In the "olden days," and I remember them well, we removed the cataract and thus rendered the eye to an "aphakic" condition (Latin for being without a lens). That resulted in elimination of the clouded lens, but was before the use of an artificial lens to replace the natural lens. The eye thus became quite farsighted usually, and thick, or strong, "aphakic spectacles," often referred to as "Coke-bottle glasses," were required. It was then obvious when a person had undergone cataract surgery. The glasses were so strong that a person could not wear the aphakic correction on one eye and regular glasses on the other eye. The aphakic spectacles caused magnification so that double vision would result. To avoid this, a contact lens could be fit on the aphakic eye. Back in those days it was usually a hard lens, and this could be quite difficult for an elderly person to handle. The usual routine was to wait until the better eye also was significantly handicapped by cataract, then do both eyes within a short interval of time. Such patients were issued temporary aphakic bifocal correction of average powers. About 6 weeks after surgery, the prescription glasses were given. Lots of patience was required by the patient. Aphakia naturally meant there was no focusing ability since the lens of the eye had been removed. Therefore, a bifocal was needed. Magnification factors of such thick lenses required periods of adjustment, as in judging size and distances. One man said his wife looked so big with his glasses on that she scared him. And of course, when the glasses were off, the vision was extremely poor. With all concerned, it obviously was quite advisable not to rush into surgery, and the phrase "waiting until the cataract was "ripe" came into practical use, mainly to give the idea of waiting for a long time.

Even considering these factors, when patients could not see, they were quite happy for visual restoration, in spite of problems with aphakia. Often, with appropriate aphakic spectacles, or contact lenses, the visual result was 20/20. One of my greatest personal satisfactions in the "old days" was a patient I operated on in a mental hospital. He was described as violent and unmanageable. He could not see, not hear, and not speak. He often charged out of his wheel chair punching "blindly" at anything within reach. When I removed his cataract, I worried because he had to be restrained postoperatively and had pus running out of his ears. On his first postoperative visit to the clinic a few days later, I put a pair of temporary aphakic glasses on him and wrote a note in large letters, saying, "Can you see?" He smiled widely and nodded yes! The poor guy had not been able to communicate, but with vision restored he became a model patient and a regular at the card table. He could also get around without a wheel chair, even without his glasses. This also reminds me of a missionary doctor I met when he returned for more training and said he did cataract surgery in Africa, with certain criteria. If natives were falling into the river or into the fire, then he would remove their cataracts. But, if they wanted to wear glasses after their surgery, then they had to go to the missionary hospital for surgery.

Well, fortunately, things have changed. For a long time now, we have used intraocular lens implants, artificial lenses to replace the extracted normal lens of the eye. Then postoperatively, a patient wears more regular glasses, such as those he or she needed before cataract development, and often much less strong than needed when younger, a form of refractive surgery. Because of this, the operated eye can work well with the unoperated eye, as before cataract development. As result, we no longer have to a wait for patient to go so blind before offering cataract surgery. That is good, because sometimes it takes years before the other eye needs surgery. With the artificial lens in place, the eye is said to be "pseudophakic," and not aphakic, as would have been without the artificial lens.

How the first artificial lens was "invented" is an interesting story. Supposedly, in London during World War II, a medical student was observing cataract surgery and was told by the ophthalmologist surgeon that the eye would be rendered aphakic by removing the lens of the eye. Being naive, but not stupid, the medical student asked why a lens could not be put back into the eye to replace the normal lens. The surgeon chuckled at the thought, because the idea of an artificial lens would bring to mind a heavy glass lens, too heavy to be tolerated. Then he recalled RAF pilots injured from plastic foreign bodies from polymethylmethacrilate canopy hoods of fighter planes damaged in dogfights over London. Such foreign body particles in the eye were found to be relatively inert, and were often tolerated to the point that destructive removal attempts could be avoided. The resultant initial plastic intraocular lenses of this material were unfortunately poorly manufactured and polished, so that most eyes receiving these lenses did not survive.

Therefore, the first artificial lenses were considered failures, and there was an interval of many years before renewed interest, and finally success (1970s). Because of concern for long-term tolerance by the eye, initial intraocular lenses were only used on the very elderly, because it was felt they would not live long enough to suffer long term complications. However, the eventual long-term success has resulted in the fact that intraocular lenses are now used even in children. The newest "IOL's" are foldable and can be inserted through a small incision requiring no stitches. What an advance from the "old-old days," even before my time, when sutures were not even available for eye surgery, and patients had to be kept in bed for days or weeks so as to not disturb their surgery wound, with both eyes patched and the head splinted by sand bags.

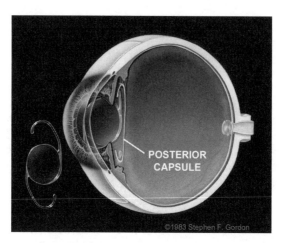

This shows the position of the intraocular lens in replacement of the normal lens of the eye (cataract), and shows the relative size of the plastic-like lens replacement. Note that the posterior capsule membrane is behind the IOL, and separates it from the vitreous cavity. Copyright © 1983 Stephen F. Gordon.

Cataract surgery has become the most frequent operation performed, and this may always be so, unless some other age-related problem requiring surgery emerges. Life expectancy is increasing, and the only way to avoid cataracts is to not get older. Some of us, of course, would have to be in our hundreds before our cataracts become very bad. Ones needs will govern whether cataract surgery is indicated. Someone who is very old, doesn't care or know how to read, sleeps most of the time, and so on, may not appreciate the improved vision. However, there is no such thing as being too old for cataract surgery. It is done under local sedated anesthesia and is not difficult to undergo healthwise. So, if people are unable to do what they wish to do visually, and are limited in vision due to cataracts, then surgery will help.

The cataract operation, like many things in medicine, has evolved tremendously in the last forty years. It has always technically been among the most difficult surgical procedures, but skill levels have progressed proportionately with the new technology. An incision or capsulotomy is made in the anterior capsule of the lens, ultrasound is used to break up the lens, and then the lens material is aspirated (sucked up). The inventor of this procedure, Dr. Charles Kelman, recently died. He has been honored as responsible for this landmark innovation in cataract surgery.

A laser is not routinely used in removal of a cataract, though the use of ultrasound is commonly confused with use of a laser. Use of a laser may follow cataract surgery, as a "touch-up" for what is sometimes called a "secondary cataract." The posterior capsule, the covering membrane of the original lens of the eye that is left in place for the artificial intraocular lens to fit into place, may become clouded, and if left unattended, it causes decreased vision, as if the cataract has come back. The "touch-up" amounts to focusing a YAG laser on the clouded posterior capsule, popping a hole through it, like a pupil behind the artificial lens, which allows light to reach the retina unobstructed. It is quick, is painless, and requires no loss of regular activity. The visual improvement is usually immediate.

An unfortunate side effect of the fact that cataract surgery has become so slick and quick, is that the procedure has become somewhat "trivialized" by high-volume cataract surgeons. The fact that such surgeons can do so many cases in half a day has made reimbursement agencies, such as Medicare and HMOs, to think that the surgical fee should be cut to a minimum. Though this may seem an advantage to the consumer, the low reimbursement has meant that a lot of cataract surgeons question the merits for themselves of doing cataract surgery, unless a high volume is available.

The high volume cataract surgeon may also not be interested in giving general care, including giving the postoperative care required, leading to "co-management" services provided postoperatively by the referring doctor. The referring doctor may be another ophthalmologist or an optometrist. To put things in proper financial perspective, a cataract surgeon has been quoted as saying that when he does cataract removal on a dog, with his veterinarian son present, he was paid $2,300. But for a human, he is paid $650 (by Medicare). I imagine he has a deal with his son for comangement.

After cataract surgery, with intraocular lens implant, a person may see quite well without glasses. However, glasses are required to see best. If a relative bilateral good distance vision is obtained, then reading glasses are required. When you think about it, there is no focusing capability of the standard rigid intraocular lens implant, but most cataract patients are old enough that they had already lost their focusing capability, and are accustomed to need something different for distance than reading, like a bifocal of trifocal. Monovision also may be created by cataract surgery, since it is possible with cataract surgery by preoperative measurements to obtain many of the goals of contact lenses or refractive surgery. Preoperative ultrasound measurements can allow the surgeon to insert an intraocular lens implant of such power that one eye can see well at distance, and the other eye better for reading. A nearsighted person can be made to see well for distance, or be at least be less nearsighted. Therefore, if people have any sign of cataract, it is probably better to not have refractive surgery, but to wait until they are ready to have their cataract removed. However, when I am told that someone, like "grandma," can see without glasses after cataract surgery, I say that she may be seeing so much better since her cataracts are removed, that she is just "showing off." Such a person may also have some monovision, so that she can see fairly well for both distance and near, but would see even better with glasses. And guess what, new intraocular lenses have become available, which allow multiple focus, so as to allow independence from glasses, often better than before cataract surgery. These will be discussed in Chapter 16, with presbyopia surgery.

10

GLAUCOMA

Another age-related common eye problem is glaucoma, affecting 4 percent of the population and increasing in frequency after age forty, with higher incidence in blacks than whites. The more common type of glaucoma is called "open angle glaucoma" and also described as the "sneak thief in the night." This is because that by the time one becomes aware of vision loss due to glaucoma, the glaucoma is usually advanced, and unfortunately the vision cannot be recovered. Vision preservation requires early detection and is one of the primary reasons to recommend routine eye examinations for health reasons, every two years after age forty.

The usual screening test that suggests glaucoma is the intraocular pressure measurement. This is only one test, however, and does not replace a complete eye examination. The usual range of "normal" intraocular pressure is from 10–22 (millimeters of mercury), but this is an average range, and in accuracy depends on who is doing the test, which method is being used for the test, and other factors, such as if the cornea of the eye is thinner than normal. And each individual is different, so that what is normal for some is not necessarily normal for others. There are those with pressures of 28 who never get glaucoma, and there are those with pressures of 16 who have glaucoma. If the pressure is 30 or more, it is usually just a matter of time before glaucoma vision loss develops. Suggestive signs of glaucoma, including a pressure above 22, cupping of the optic nerve, or vision loss not otherwise explained, suggest the need for further testing for glaucoma. A visual field test, testing peripheral vision with computerized technique, can detect earliest sign of glaucoma. Also new optic nerve fiber photographic techniques help early diagnosis and follow-up. Even with all these test techniques, the diagnosis is often not easy. Treatment principles have varied from lowering all suspiciously high intraocular pressures, in spite of the possibility of treating some who will never get glaucoma, versus requiring confirmation of diagnosis via visual field exam and other factors before treating.

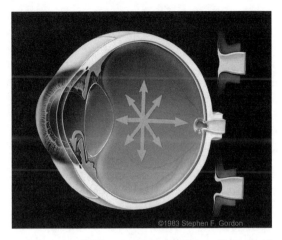

An arrow shows flow of aqueous fluid through the pupil and into the anterior chamber angle trabecular meshwork for drainage. It also shows expansive arrows suggesting increased intraocular pressure and the resulting cupping of the optic nerve, compared to the small cross-section of relatively flat and "perfectly" normal optic nerve. Some cupping of the nerve is often normal with nearsightedness, but is less commonly normal in farsightedness. Copyright © 1983 Stephen F. Gordon.

Visual field (peripheral or side vision) loss from glaucoma is usually not noted by the patient until often too late. Peripheral vision loss can be insidious and sneaky. Typically, glaucomatous loss of vision may be toward the nose, where it may not be noticed. Loss of central or reading vision may not develop until quite late in the disease, so that a person may be able to see 20/20, but not be able to maneuver through a room of furniture without falling down. This may be called "tunnel vision," though there is no such thing, since one's side vision expands with increased distance, like a cheerleaders megaphone, no matter how bad it is restricted. But the term implies correctly problems in mobility.

As time goes on, open angle glaucoma is felt more and more to be a unique disease of the optic nerve, so that some people have optic nerves more sensitive to pressure than others. Cupping of the optic nerve can suggest glaucoma, even if the eye pressures are relatively low. A flat optic nerve is easily described as normal, but a bowing backward of the optic nerve centrally, called cupping, to some degree can also be normal. When the whole optic nerve is cupped, or scooped out like a big bowl, advanced glaucoma is pretty obvious. Vertically oval cups of significant size, as compared to horizontally oval cups, especially if recorded as enlarging over a period of time, suggest glaucoma. POAG (primary open angle glaucoma) may be one-eyed in onset, but involvement of both eyes is highly suspected eventually.

Open angle glaucoma is diagnosed, compared to narrow angle glaucoma, by gonioscopy. The gonioscope is a special mirrored contact-lens-type device that allows visualization in the anterior chamber angles, the space between the root of the pupil forming iris tissue and the peripheral cornea. It is like looking around corners. Latticelike tissue called meshwork can be seen if the angle is "open." The meshwork filters and allows drainage of aqueous fluid that is being constantly replaced and circulating through the pupil. In open angles glaucoma, the problem seems comparable to a plumbing problem, whereby the fluid does not drain properly. Then back-up pressure results in the eye, as if the meshwork is not letting the fluid filter through properly, resulting in increased intraocular back pressure. Another comparison, is like a rubber tire that becomes overinflated. In the case of the eye, the rigid sclera prevents stretching, but the weak point is the optic nerve, and this is where the damage occurs.

The treatment of chronic open angle glaucoma is usually eye drops, which lower the intraocular pressure by either decreasing the amount of aqueous fluid formed, or by promoting better drainage of the waterlike aqueous, or a combination of both. There are many eye drops for glaucoma, new ones appearing often. Side effects and cost may affect choice of drops. The effectiveness can vary per individual, so that changes may need be made, and sometimes two or three kinds of drops may be necessary to keep the pressure in safe ranges. Once treatment is begun, it usually needs to be continued indefinitely. Patient compliance is required, including follow-up exams. One is not able to "feel" if the pressure is getting higher, unless the pressure rises rapidly, or is quite high. Then, the pain is not in the eye itself, but rather in the eyebrow.

Success of treatment is gauged by significant lowering of the eye pressure, but better confirmed by fact that visual field defects, previously noted, do not worsen. It should not be expected that vision, including visual field defects will improve. The main goal is one of holding the line, such that further worsening of the visual field is not happening. Other factors are monitoring the appearance of the optic nerve, the cupping, and nerve fiber tests that also can detect loss of function. So I tell patients not to expect their eyes to seem better while being treated, since they are unaware usually of the visual field defect in the first place. Don't expect to see better or feel like the eyes feel better. Don't expect to be able to judge whether the pressure is lower, you can't feel it. What the patient needs to do is follow instructions, take the medicine, and be good about follow-up examinations.

Treatment with eye drops is considered preferable to laser or surgery methods, as long as successful, due to lesser potential complications. Laser treatment amounts to making burn spots in the angular meshwork, to promoted better drainage of fluid and therefore lower intraocular pressure. The main complication, is that the effect may be unsuccessful, just temporary, or only partially successful. Newer lasers are available, but long-term beneficial effect remains to be seen, and laser treatment has not, so far, replaced eye drops as primary treatment. Faced with the inconvenience of continued need for use of eye drops, some patients are attracted to the "quick fix" potential of laser trabeculoplasty, but unfortunately close follow-up is required so as to not ignore eventual failure of the procedure. Such patients may need eye drops again or repeat laser treatment.

Surgical treatment of glaucoma is usually reserved for glaucoma patients whose pressures are not controlled by eye drops, or laser trabeculoplasty. The surgery provides a "filter," or surgically created extra pathway for the aqueous fluid to drain from the eye, so as to lower the intraocular pressure. Success is common, but not guaranteed. Complications include failure to filter, infection, or cataract. If a cataract is already present, a combination of cataract surgery and glaucoma filtering procedure may be performed. Another potential complication is that what may ordinarily be a simple conjunctivitis may spread to involve the inside of the eye, and become a more serious endophthalmitis. Fortunately, this is a rare complication.

Other surgical treatment of glaucoma can involve an artificial implant or valve, which helps regulate fluid drainage from the eye, often with great success. Endocyclophotocoagulation can also be performed, involving laser microscopic treatments on the ciliary body. This is considered as optimum in timing, to do during phakoemulsification in cataract surgery, in patients who are controlled by their glaucoma medications, in hopes of avoiding glaucoma drops.

The idea of a quick fix for glaucoma is not new, but not universally accepted. In other words, there are those who have said, let's go directly to laser or surgical control of intraocular pressure, rather than all the bother of using eye drops. It is true that the cumulative effects of using eye drops indefinitely can amount to significant expense, so that procedures, if they work, cannot seem so expensive, in the long run. This is the problem, because the combination of lack of success, requiring resumed use of eye drops anyway, and the potential complications including cataracts and infection following filtering surgery, makes the use of eye drops not so expensive, after all.

As an interesting side story, I once had a patient from England, who was referred while living there to the ophthalmic surgeon for suspicion of glaucoma. The doctor just happened to be doing his "surgery day," and just added her to his schedule. He performed bilateral filtering procedures, apparently successfully. She did not show signs of glaucoma when I examined her, nor any complication from the surgery. But, of course, we do not know if she had glaucoma in the first place, since she did not have proper testing.

Acute angle closure glaucoma is less common, but potentially more dramatic in cause of sudden loss of vision. As disclosed by gonioscopy, if the space between the base of the iris, the colored part, and the peripheral cornea is too narrow, then aqueous fluid cannot drain properly, resulting in potentially a sudden rise in intraocular pressure. The incidence of narrow angles anatomically is about 2 percent in whites, whereas the incidence of angle closure glaucoma is less than 0.1 percent. The highest incidence is in Eskimos. The potential of angle closure glaucoma is greatly increased in small, farsighted eyes. Acute angle closure glaucoma attack is the usual first sign of the problem. Pain results, contrary to more common open angle glaucoma, not in the eye as may be expected, but in the eye brow on that side, due to sudden rise in eye pressure.

Sequence of events in acute angle closure then can include redness of the eye, blurred vision, photosensitivity, nausea and vomiting. The pupil becomes enlarged. Occurrence of such attacks have happened postoperatively in general surgery, when atropine-like medications having pupil dilating side effects have been used as part of anesthesia, and the nausea and vomiting symptoms often have diverted attention from angle closure glaucoma attack of the eye to some sort of abdominal problem. Dilating the pupil can potentially trigger an attack, but this does not happen very often in the course of eye examination. For one thing, if the anterior chamber angle looks narrow, then electively it is decided often not to dilate the pupil.

Cold medications containing pupil dilating decongestant drugs can precipitate an attack, and this is the reason for the warning on such products, if one reads the fine print. However, the difference between the danger for open angle glaucoma, the most common kind of glaucoma, and potential angle closure glaucoma, is not defined in the warning labels. The average open angle glaucoma patient can take cold medications without concern. It certainly is acceptable to question your eye doctor about whether it is all right to take cold medications with your kind of glaucoma.

Sometimes there are "mini attacks" of angle closure, something, if recognized, could predict eventual major attack of angle closure glaucoma. Typically, an affected person says that after watching TV at night, they get a headache, and have to go to bed before it goes away. If questioned, they usually admit that they watch TV with little or no room light and the headache is in the eyebrow region. Under these circumstances, the pupils will enlarge because the room is dark, triggering a small attack of angle closure glaucoma, not so bad as to prevent them falling to sleep. The pupils normally become smaller in sleep, and the attack can be aborted.

Treatment of an angle closure glaucoma attack is usually an emergency. Drops to constrict the pupil (miotics such as pilocarpine) are used, plus diuretic pills like Diamox, and hypertonic solutions orally taken to draw fluid from the eye. The combination must work rapidly, and within a few minutes signs of improvement can be detected. Seldom is emergency surgery required, and if the pressure is controlled by medication, it may be better to await signs of less inflammation, within the next day or so.

Whereas surgical iridectomy was once indicated, now laser iridotomy as an outpatient can be done with less trauma and inconvenience to the patient. Continued treatment with miotics may be advisable to avoid further attacks, and sometimes there is a combination of open angle and narrow angle glaucoma, such that additional glaucoma drops are required. Cataracts commonly result, following an attack of angle closure glaucoma, and may form more rapidly than age-related-type cataract.

Bilateral simultaneous attacks of angle closure glaucoma are fortunately rare, but the unaffected eye is potentially at risk in the future, due to likely anatomic similarity. The chances of an angle closure attack in the other eye are estimated as between 40 percent and 80 percent within five to ten years. Prophylactic treatment of the other eye, usually in the form of laser iridotomy is recommended. A difference of opinion may be encountered relative to need to treat "potential" angle closure glaucoma, meaning someone whose angles look narrow enough to have an attack of glaucoma. Many, perhaps most, such people would never get an attack of glaucoma, but to be on the "safe side," prophylactic treatment with pilocarpine (pupil constricting) drops or laser iridotomy may be elected, or a combination of these treatments. A provocative test, dilating the pupil to see if the pressure goes up, can help decide if prophylactic treatment is needed.

Pilocarpine is one of the original eye drops for treatment of glaucoma. As mentioned, it is now used mainly for narrow or potential narrow angle glaucoma. As a miotic, this means that the pupil is made smaller. This is especially helpful in narrow angles, as it encourages aqueous fluid drainage without obstruction, by increasing the space between the iris pupil forming tissue and the peripheral portions of the cornea. It also lowers pressure in open angle glaucoma, but is less used currently due to side effects. These side effects include eyebrow ache while getting used to the miotic drops, and change in vision. Because the pupil is smaller, less light gets through, and because it is kept small by the drops, a person has a problem adapting to the dark, as in night driving, or in going from outdoors into a movie theater. A positive side effect, however, is that, because the pupil is small, a "pinhole" effect occurs, and people on miotics are less dependent on their glasses. Another side effect desirable to some, is that the eyes appear lighter, or bluer, with small pupils, a factor considered attractive by a female patient.

There are many kinds of eye drops for open angle glaucoma control. They differ in action, affecting aqueous eye fluid inflow and outflow, or both. They all have potential undesirable side effects, though obviously not often enough to make them not useful. Nevertheless, it is necessary to determine which will work best for each individual, and trial periods are necessary. Among the most common are beta-blockers, which are cheaper, quite effective as an initial treatment, and available in generic form. But beta-blockers can also be a problem for people who have trouble with asthma or emphysema. Others include prostaglandins, androgenic drops, and cholinesterase inhibitors.

Used topically, not much of these eye drops gets into the blood stream, but obviously enough can do so, and cause systemic side effects. This can be minimized by holding two fingers, one on each side of the nose, between the eyes, in a pinching fashion for a few seconds after instilling the drops. Doing this right after using the eye drop helps keep it from running down the nose right away, where it may be rapidly absorbed into the blood stream, and also helps the eye itself absorb the medication better.

Patients need to understand that taking the glaucoma eye drops for awhile does not make the problem go away, like taking an antibiotic, it just helps prevent further damage by progression of glaucoma. Yes, this usually means for the rest of the patient's life, and unfortunately what medication seems satisfactory initially may need be replaced or added upon to continue to assure safe control in the future. The stated goal is to lower the pressure about 20 percent. Newer and better topical medications are being developed. Unfortunately, most new medications are not "generic," and insurance coverage may not provide payment. Hopefully, Plan D will help Medicare patients.

Patient compliance, the following of instructions faithfully, can be a problem. It is difficult to remember to take eye drops several times a day, so that ones once taken at bedtime or first thing in the morning are easier to remember. Newer medications include some combinations that may simplify use, many not yet available in the United States. Available in Canada are such things as Xalacom (Xalatan and timolol), Combigen (Alphagan and timolol), and Extravan (Travatan and timolol). It is also difficult to predict how much damage can be expected by missing a drop now and then. One must do the best one can, and remember to take their one's medications with them on trips, including to the hospital. The hospital may insist on giving you their own eye drops, but they will need to see what you have been taking. And by the way, when you leave the hospital, be sure to ask for the partially used bottles of medicine the hospital has been giving you. They are yours, since you paid for them.

Marijuana has been reported as having pressure lowering potential, such that is listed as a treatment of glaucoma. However, I know of no ophthalmologists prescribing this "medication."

11

MACULAR DEGENERATION

Macular degeneration affects 2–3 percent of the population. It seems to be becoming more common, because it is usually age related and people are living longer. It is commonly referred to as AMD, for age-related macular degeneration. So, like the incidence of cataracts and glaucoma, the numbers of age related macular degeneration patients will increase. However, unlike glaucoma, the incidence of AMD is higher in whites than blacks. With macular degeneration the loss of vision is central, affecting reading and color vision, but usually not affecting peripheral or side vision. If comparing eye to camera anatomically, the macula is the central point of focus on the retina of light or images entering the eye. The macula is composed of 100 percent cones, whereas the peripheral retina is more composed of rods (useful in night vision). If there is a "flaw" in the macula, then, like having a "flaw" in camera film, and no matter how well images are focused by the eye and corrective glasses, the "pictures" don't turn out right.

Though macular degeneration is generally limited to central vision, the inability to read can be so severe as to prevent passing a driver's test, and even so severe as to be considered "legally blind." This means that a person is unable to see better than 20/200, even with glasses. However, complete blindness is not expected, and the problem may always remain mild. So progression of the problem may be expected, but is not inevitable. There are even cases of spontaneous improvement to some degree. AMD is said to be the leading cause of legal blindness in the over sixty-five age group. However, even if legally blind, those with macular degeneration problems are not the ones needing a white cane. They can be expected to be able to get around as far as mobility and not need much help in self-care. Typically, they are reluctant to give up their driver's license, as they recognize little problems in driving, due to good peripheral vision. If severe, such people learn to look to one side to see better, for example, to look at one's ear to be able to see the nose. Therefore, they sometimes seem to not look other people "in the eye" when talking to them.

The central macula is composed of 100 percent cones, and is so sensitive as to be able to differentiate a 1-degree angular interval at 20 feet, hence 20/20 vision. A mixture with "rods" develops gradually away from the macula, until, eventually, in the peripheral retina, there are mainly rods. What this means is that loss of the central or reading vision is due to damage to the cones in the macula, and damage to peripheral or night vision is due to damage to the rods, as in retinitis pigmentosa. So there are worse things to happen to one's vision than macular degeneration. For one thing, since AMD is age related, people with macular degeneration have usually enjoyed good vision for most of their life, and they also do not become totally blind. Comparatively, those with retinitis pigmentosa may have problems at an early age, involving loss of night and peripheral vision, and may eventually lose their central vision also, so as to become almost totally blind. Also severe glaucoma can cause more complete blindness so as to be worse in comparison.

AMD may complicate the diagnosis of glaucoma or cataract effect on vision, other age-related potential problems. It may be difficult to separate one problem from the other as to the percentage of effect on vision. This issue is especially important in determining if or when cataract surgery should be performed, since minimal improvement of vision postoperatively would be disappointing. Improvement of vision with a pinhole test, demonstrating better vision than with glasses, may be reassuring that the problem is mainly cataract. Another test is the Amsler grid, which is a page with small squares and a dot in the center. With AMD, the lines around the central dot become crooked and distorted, and the dot in the center may be absent. Sometimes, the effect of other problems is not fully evident until after cataract surgery, and removing the cataract may subsequently improve intraocular exam so that other problems may be better evaluated. However, unfortunately, cataract surgery may also stimulate macular degeneration to become worse, as well as diabetic retinopathy. These are factors that suggest a conservative approach to cataract surgery, especially if the cataract is not so dense as to obstruct adequate examination of the retina.

There are different types of macular degeneration, but most are age related. Hereditary forms occur and usually result in earlier development of the problem. A common situation occurs when spots are visible in the "macula" upon routine eye examination, called drusen. Too often the statement is made that a person has macular degeneration because of these spots. However, measurable loss of vision must be present before macular degeneration should be diagnosed. The presence of drusen spots often anticipates or represents an early sign of impending macular degeneration, but vision may continue to be normal. On the other hand, diagnostic signs of macular degeneration may be sometimes so difficult to see upon retinal examination, that though macular degeneration is suspected, special tests are required, such as flourescein angiography, to confirm the diagnosis. This test may also help determine if the type of macular degeneration is "wet" or "dry."

The dry form accounts for about 90 percent of patients with AMD. However, the wet type of macular degeneration, associated with neovascularization, or new blood vessel formation, accounts for about 90 percent of cases of severe vision loss due to AMD. In general there are few treatment alternatives for the dry type, and many new treatments are now available for the wet form of AMD. So quite often you may hear about a new treatment for macular degeneration in the news, and these are usually for the wet form. The plenitude has resulted due to the failure of most procedures to give much success in the past.

A study recently showed that vitamins containing zinc and lutein may help decrease progression of dry macular degeneration, and are recommended for this reason. However, taking such pills may not be expected to avoid macular degeneration in those destined to have it, or improve vision in those who have lost vision due to macular degeneration. There are many different brands containing about the same combinations of vitamins, zinc, and lutein. No one brand is outstanding, though one label, from Allergan, was involved in the study from which all get their encouragement. All are over-the-counter drugs, which is good for availability, but perhaps bad in that any medical insurance coverage does not apply. Another problem is that the uninformed may be taking these medicines unnecessarily, in attempt to make their eyes better.

A patient recently informed me that her relative in Canada is undergoing rheophoresis for macular degeneration. This apparently is a form of plasmaphoresis, whereby blood is drawn from a patient, the plasma is separated, and certain proteins and lipoproteins are filtered from the blood before returning it into the patient. Though some good results are reported, it is only experimental in this country, and the fact that these elements reappear in the blood rapidly makes this form of treatment questionable in theory.

Treatment of wet macular degeneration is best performed by retinal disease specialists in ophthalmology. Utilizing a photographic technique called flourescein angiography, they can determine whether they are dealing with the dry or wet form of AMD. Thus they can visualize the subretinal leaking of fluid and new blood vessel formation, called neovascularization, in the wet form. These new vessels are delicate and unhealthy, and can rupture and bleed spontaneously. This bleeding results in scar formation, destroying retinal function. Of course, in the delicate macula, the result can be disastrous in visual effect and be sudden in onset.

Different approaches have been taken to treat the wet form of macular degeneration. Utilizing a laser, spot treatment of leaking or potential leaks from vessels can be done. However, the laser burn creates a scar, and if this involves the macula near the center, the vision is reduced, even if it is relatively successful in reducing the chance of new vessel formation. A newer laser treatment is photo dynamic therapy, which utilizes a more superficial treatment better directed to areas that need treatment. Visudyne, a photosensitive drug, is injected intravenously, and then a low, insensitive nonthermal laser is used to destroy neovascularization, with little scarring. Results have been an improvement over regular laser treatment, but often not good enough.

The most drastic surgical treatment is called macular translocation. This involves moving or translocating the retina so that the choroidal neovascularization is no longer under the fovea, and can be treated later. Complications include seeing less well than hoped and this form of surgery is used for those whose vision is so bad that they are desperate to regain even a little vision. Another procedure, not yet approved by the Food and Drug Administration, is the IMT, or implantable miniature telescope, which is placed in the lens capsule after removing the lens, instead of the conventional intraocular lens implant. This has allowed improvement of vision in volunteers of a few lines on the Snellen chart, but there is concern about approval, due to a high loss of endothelial cells of the cornea, meaning perhaps significant future complications.

Even more recent has been the treatment of wet macular degeneration by means of injecting drugs that discourage neovascularization, some of which have originated in use as anticancer medications. These drugs, such as macugen, avastin, and lucentis, are actually injected through the sclera into the vitreous of the eye. There have been some good results, including reports of improvement of vision in the case of avastin and lucentis, whereas macugen has been more for maintenance, to avoid worsening. "Implants" of such materials are being tried so as to avoid the need for such frequent injections.

The most common type of macular degeneration, the dry type, cannot be treated by laser. The process seems to be more of a lack of nutrition or withering away of cells, related to age in most part, but certainly not inevitable in the majority of the aged. Laser treatment would only do more damage in an area that is quite delicate. Some have suggested that the dry form of macular degeneration is just an earlier form of the wet type. My clinical observation suggests that they are two different processes, both with potentially disastrous effects, but that the wet type carries with it the threat of sudden irreversible vision loss.

The natural course of macular degeneration is to become worse, but this is not inevitable, and progression may be quite slow. Unfortunately, especially in the wet or neovascular type, there may be sudden worsening. There are typically "good days" and "bad days" for those with macular degeneration, and general variation of vision, affected by lighting and time of day. Enjoy the "good days," if you have macular degeneration. If the vision gets worse, it is not the patient's fault from trying to read or using the eyes too much. The best one can do is to seek good professional advice. If a patient wants to explore all avenues, we of course first send them to a retinal specialist. Routine examinations, every two years after age forty, are recommended. If the vision is normal, then there is no macular degeneration, even with a family history of the problem. If the vision is not normal, and another reason cannot be found, then a retinal specialist may be consulted. However, even though concerned due to a family history of macular degeneration, it is not necessary or practical for all such people to be seen by a retinal specialist for a routine examination.

There are other less common problems that can affect central or reading vision, and which can be confused with macular degeneration, but may involve different forms of treatment. Cystoid macular edema is an occasional complication of cataract surgery, which can be transient and can be treated. A macular "hole" can develop spontaneously, even in younger age. The degree of visual defect from this can vary, and surgery may be recommended in severe cases. Macular hole is usually monocular, and is not the source of a retinal detachment, like which can result from holes elsewhere in the retina. Also, a membrane may grow over the macula, called an epiretinal membrane or cellophane retinopathy, spontaneously or as a result of inflammation in the eye. Treatment depends on severity of affect on vision, and involves surgical removal of the vitreous (vitrectomy), with peeling the membrane off the retina microscopically. Complete recovery cannot be guaranteed, but spontaneous recovery is not unknown. Central serous retinopathy affects young males, and is described in Chapter 14.

The hereditary involvement in macular degeneration is an area of intense research, with some interesting results. The genetic localization of the problem raises questions as to etiology, and also questions about eventual gene therapy. This certainly would be a big reward to those involved in such research, but seems to be something not foreseen in the near future.

PART IV
SPECIAL CONSIDERATIONS

12

VISUAL AIDS

Subnormal vision can be helped by "visual aids." These are mainly magnifying devices, often aided by good lighting. Some good variations include large-screen magnifying TV or computer monitors, which can be used to read letters and books. There are special methods to aid in walking and the use of seeing-eye dogs. Special courses and aids can help in self-care, cooking, and computer use. The Braille Society is good for evaluating people with acquired adult vision loss for visual aids, which is usually a trial-and-error process, and not just to teach Braille. It is actually quite difficult for someone to learn Braille if the person once had fairly good vision, especially an adult. There is a huge difference between being "legally blind" from something like macular degeneration, when usually one can care for themselves, and someone whose vision is so poor as to qualify for a seeing-eye dog.

There is often confusion about the limitation of glasses in helping those with poor vision. One may think that it should be possible to make glasses as strong as a magnifying glass. However, the more the magnification, the closer one has to hold things to be in focus, and people don't like holding reading material up to their nose. Usual full-strength reading glasses, required by those of us in our sixties and beyond, and taking into account that distance vision is either good or corrected by glasses, are +2.5 diopters. This allows those with normal vision to read small print at 1/4 meter or 16 inches, and this is closer than many would like to have to hold things. For subnormal vision, a +3 may be tolerated, with a focal distance of 1/3 meter (13 inches), or at most a +4 with about a 10-inch working distance. However, more magnification to allow seeing small print may not be tolerable, because of having to hold things too close.

Blindness from congenital reasons is tragic, but apparently not so bad as congenital deafness in retarding learning. There are, of course, degrees of visual handicap, and many children with visual problems can get through primary education fairly well, with assistance. The print in children's books is usually relatively large, and this helps. The computer age has probably helped also, by presenting larger print. Most states have special education facilities for the blind. In my home state of Iowa, there is a school for the blind. Larger states have local special primary schools with special facilities for those with a visual handicap. I was impressed by a statement made by the school nurse at the Iowa School for the Blind. She described a sort of caste system based on how well a child could see. The "Sight Savers" were children who had some vision, at least enough to get around. The "Brailles" were children with little or no vision. Being a Sight Saver apparently resulted in a leadership status, each Sight Saver leading one or two Brailles, between classes, to their next assignment. However, she pointed out that the Brailles were the better students. They accepted their problem and learned Braille so as to become educated. The Sight Savers too often apparently tried to fool others, and as a result mainly themselves, into thinking that they could do the school work without learning Braille.

Telescopic lenses are available as a distance aid for help with movies or theater. There are even such telescopic aids for driving a car, approved in some states, but these can be quite dangerous due to restricted side vision. Another practical point is that those blinded, for whatever reason, still want to wear their glasses. True, the glasses may be of little, if any, help. Nevertheless, blind people who are used to wearing glasses will often want to continue to do so. Their glasses need to be upgraded when worn out, even if it is a matter of duplicating what they have been wearing. They may feel almost naked without the glasses, and the glasses probably do give some visual aid in certain cases.

Among the most dramatic visual aids available are the TV and the computer, whereby print can be so enlarged that a person with limited vision can read a letter or pay bills. I have heard of a Microsoft program called Zoom Text, which can enlarge print, but more importantly has also a program whereby what appears on the printed page can be read aloud, called Doc (document) Reader. Such visual aids are rather expensive but greatly appreciated.

Some patients ask, "Well, doctor, why can't you just transplant me a new eye?" I reply that the eye is like brain tissue, that we will be able to transplant eyes about when we become able to transplant brains, and that we have a really long list of people who need a new brain. Low-vision specialists are available among ophthalmologists and optometrists, who can work with people visually disabled.

13

Diabetes

Diabetes mellitus is type I if insulin is required, and type II if controlled by oral medication or diet (non-insulin-dependent). In both types, complications involving the eyes can occur, though more likely with type I. Rarely, but sometimes, eye exam can trigger the diagnosis. For example, becoming nearsighted rather rapidly, when not being so before, can be due to high blood sugar. Then, when insulin treatment is utilized, following diagnosis, a shift toward an unusual degree of farsightedness can occur. Certainly, when the refractive error or need for glasses is bouncing around, it is best to postpone a change in glasses until the blood sugar is stabilized. I have even seen such a shift occur following rapid weight loss involved in treating diabetes, but generally the blood sugar shift causing a change in vision due to need for a change in glasses is related to type I, or insulin insulin-required, diabetes. In terms of the discovery of diabetes, it is also sometimes true that the discovery of posterior subcapsular cataract in a younger-than-usual patient, can suggest latent diabetes, as I have experienced with a few patients who were told by me to get tested for diabetes. Otherwise, the eye doctor is not usually the first to diagnose diabetes.

The usual reason to advise diabetics of all types to get annual eye examinations is to look for what is called diabetic retinopathy. Diabetic retinopathy amounts to stereotypical retinal hemorrhages and exudates, or macular edema. These have such a unique appearance as to suggest diabetes, without a history. There may also be a vitreous hemorrhages resulting from diabetes. Usually it takes seven to ten years before retinopathy occurs, and when evident sooner, it may suggest the patient was diabetic longer than suspected. Such retinopathy can be treated with laser to avoid progress. Fortunately diabetic retinopathy is not inevitable. Naturally, it can be assumed that good control of diabetes lessens the chance of retinopathy, but unfortunately there is no guarantee of immunity from retinopathy in diabetics. Treatment of associated hypertension may also diminish chances of diabetic retinopathy.

Diabetic retinopathy can accompany other eye diseases, and can make it difficult to gauge the severity of each component of the visual problem. For example, diabetics get involvement of the macula, and special testing may be necessary to exclude macular degeneration of other origin. Also, cataracts are common, either the age-related variety or the type caused by diabetes. The obscuring of the inside of the eye due to cataracts may make it difficult to evaluate the degree of retinopathy, as well as to perform needed laser treatments. So even if we are not sure that cataract is the main cause of loss of vision, a better ability to evaluate the retina for diabetic retinopathy with clearer view following cataract extraction may be expected. Complicating the decision for surgery, however, is the known fact that diabetic retinopathy frequently takes a change for the worse following cataract surgery. Considering all the factors, and presenting them to the patient, is one of the major jobs of the operating ophthalmologist.

14

NEUROLOGIC CONDITIONS AFFECTING VISION

The eye is a neurosensory organ, an extension of the brain. It can be affected by many neurosensory or neurological diseases.

CAUSES OF SUDDEN VISION LOSS

Vascular Occlusion

Vascular occlusion can be of the central artery or vein or branches of these. If central, meaning the main large artery entering or the large vein leaving the eye, vision loss is severe, and the prognosis is poor for regaining useful vision. It is sometimes called a "stroke" of the eye, properly suggesting the fact that it has to do with circulation of the eye which can suddenly be closed off, as in a brain-attack-type stroke, and that function may not return. Of course, it is limited to the eye, so do not put on a driver's license form that you had a stroke following such an episode, or they may deny the license even when the other eye sees well. In central retinal vein thrombosis, secondary glaucoma may develop within ninety days, which can be painful and difficult to treat. Recovery of vision loss may occur in branch vessel occlusion, meaning that only a branch of the main vessel is involved. Sometimes, a plaque of cholesterol can be seen blocking an artery, and this suggests carotid artery disease on that side. This finding, of course, is quite significant. A stroke affecting the brain could occur later since the presence of the plaque in the eye suggests that another plaque could in the future break off from the main carotid artery to block a vessel in the brain.

Transient vision loss, from above or below, as if a window blind is drawn and then again retracted, is called *amaurosis fugax*. This suggests carotid artery disease and could warn of potential vascular occlusion in one eye, or, as mentioned, even a stroke. If you get such symptoms of transient vision loss, you should see your eye doctor.

Ischemic Optic Neuropathy

Ischemic optic neuropathy (ION) is a problem occurring usually in older people, especially those with hypertensive arteriosclerotic vascular disease, or diabetics, whereby sudden loss of vision can occur to a noticeable degree, or even almost complete loss of vision. It is painless and without warning. Typically, visual field testing may show loss of the upper or lower half of vision, but field loss may vary to even complete extinguishing of vision. Prognosis is poor for visual recovery, and though we do not understand the mechanism of the loss of vision, we know that the other eye may be at risk at some future date. Nonarteritic ischemic optic neuropathy (NAION) is the term used to describe ION, as compared with temporal arteritis, which is inflammatory and, therefore, arteritic. This term, NAION, is used in reference to a discussion of the sudden loss of vision associated with the use of Viagra and other such medicines. NAION usually occurs within a short interval (hours) after using such medications, if due to such use, and should warn that the problem may occur in the other eye should there be continued use of the medicine.

Temporal Arteritis

Temporal arteritis is also called cranial arteritis and causes arteritic optic neuropathy. The signs affecting the eye involve sudden vision loss associated usually with tenderness of the temporal artery area on that side of the head, and often jaw ache. There may be headaches also, and other serious neurological complications can follow, since other arteries in the brain can be involved. Diagnosis can be highly suggested by the elevated sedimentation rate of blood and confirmed by a temporal artery biopsy. Temporal arteritis needs treatment with oral steroids, often on an emergency basis. Some visual recovery may occur, but the chief reason for urgent treatment is to protect the other eye, and of course to avoid life-threatening complications. The reason for the term cranial arteritis is that other vessels in the brain are likely involved. A sedimentation rate test of blood can predict how active or severe is the problem and is used as a sign of success of treatment, acutely and for long-term management. The use of oral steroids can then be titrated according to the sedimentation rate, and if it shows signs of rising again, the oral steroids can be resumed.

Optic Neuritis

Optic neuritis can be from various causes, but the most common and striking example is associated with multiple sclerosis (MS). In fact, this may present as the first symptom of MS and, therefore, in younger people. Vision may be severely and suddenly lost but usually also recovers in part, or almost completely. Usually only one eye is involved in the initial attack. Recovery can occur spontaneously but is aided by corticosteroid treatment. Intravenous steroids are preferred to oral, having to do with lessening of the potential development of other symptoms. Treatment and confirmation of diagnosis is best managed by a neurologist. In years past, early diagnosis of MS was one of exclusion, meaning that the suspicion is high, but no tests can confirm. Now magnetic resonance imaging (MRI) tests of the brain can detect plaques, suggesting MS as a positive diagnosis. Visual field abnormalities may disappear, with the only late sign being paleness of the optic nerve, something that may be overlooked, without history.

Vitreous Hemorrhage

Vitreous hemorrhage is often spontaneous and may be from a cause unknown. It is not a neurology problem, but is one of the causes of sudden loss of vision. Depending on the severity of hemorrhage, vision may be clouded partially, or almost completely blacked out. However, such hemorrhage may also be part of a retinal tear leading to retinal detachment, or, more commonly, a complication of diabetes. If mild or uncomplicated, the vitreous hemorrhage can spontaneously clear with time. If severe, or if accompanying retinal detachment, the blood can be removed by vitrectomy surgery. As true of other causes, such sudden loss of vision demands urgent examination by an eye doctor.

OTHER NEUROLOGICAL PROBLEMS

There are a great many neurological problems that manifest themselves in eye symptoms, and here are a few more.

Optic Nerve Problems

The optic nerve, cranial nerve II, like other cranial nerves, originates directly from the brain, as a forward extension of the brain. Swelling of the optic nerve can be due to papilledema, papillitis, or pseudopapilledema. True papilledema, a swelling of the optic nerve, visible in an intraocular eye examination, may signify increased intracranial pressure from various causes. For example, it can occur after an injury involving intracranial hemorrhage, or a brain tumor. It can also occur in a more benign condition called pseudotumor cerebri. Papillitis is a swelling of the optic nerve due to inflammation. Differential diagnosis involves the fact that vision is usually reduced with papillitis, whereas it is often normal with papilledema. Also, a visual field test will usually show a central defect with papillitis, and may be normal except for an enlarged blind spot with papilledema.

There can be a variation of the appearance of the optic nerve. For example, farsighted people typically have flat to slightly swollen-appearing optic nerves. Pseudochoke is a term used for situations where the optic nerve appears swollen, but actually is not. One cause of a pseudochoke is drusen of the optic nerve, benign cystic bulges, which can cause swelling of the optic nerve, and usually do not affect vision, though some sign can be demonstrated in visual field testing. In the exam, the appearance of spontaneous venous pulsation on the nerve can reassure that there is no increased intracranial pressure. But unfortunately it is not uniform that a pulsation of the vein is normally present, and it would take information from a former exam to prove that the pulsation had been changed from spontaneous pulsation to no pulsation.

The optic nerve is probably most commonly involved in open-angle glaucoma, where, in recent theory, the main problem of the disease suggests unusual sensitivity of the optic nerve to intraocular pressure. The result is the opposite of swelling of the nerve; the optic nerve actually becomes "cupped" or excavated. Here also, however, there is great variation, which can be normal. For example, contrary to farsighted people who usually have flat-appearing optic nerves, nearsighted people usually have some cupping of the nerve. Change in cupping noted on repeat exams is quite significant in suggesting the need for testing for glaucoma, even with lower intraocular pressure.

The optic nerve, like other cranial nerves, comes directly from the brain. Therefore, claims made, as in the past, by chiropractors, that spinal adjustment can help the eyes, are totally not supported anatomically.

Multiple Sclerosis (MS)

Sometimes eye symptoms are the first signs of MS; about one-third of MS patients present with optic neuritis as the first sign. About 50 percent of MS patients will develop optic neuritis. Sudden vision loss in a younger patient, typically a woman in her thirties, in one eye, can be the first symptom of MS, called retrobulbar neuritis. It is called retrobulbar because the nerve swelling is behind the eye, and therefore does not cause visible swelling of the nerve. Ocular signs include reduced vision, visual field defect, and what is called an afferent pupil defect (the pupil does not react normally to light).

Spontaneous improvement can be expected from retrobulbar neuritis due to MS, even return to normal vision and return to normal visual field test in about 85 percent of patients. The only lasting sign may be a slight paleness of the optic nerve appearance. The use of steroids may speed up recovery, but recent reports suggest that such treatment may lead to other symptoms more quickly than if spontaneous improvement is allowed to happen. It is helpful for a neurologist to make this decision, and to interpret other tests such as an MRI. An MRI can help establish diagnosis of early MS. Later, in most cases unfortunately, other signs of MS can appear to confirm the diagnosis. A neurologist may use immunomudulatory agents specific for MS to reduce the number and severity of eventual episodes.

Double Vision (Diplopia)

Double vision may not be from a serious cause, especially if of long duration and controllable by prisms in glasses. However, images close together are much more annoying than images more separated so as to enable to concentrate on just one of the images with less confusion. Neurological causes are multiple, including stroke, MS, or myasthenia gravis. Often the cause is due to "ischemia," or cause unknown, followed by spontaneous recovery. The cause of ischemia could be diabetes, hypertension, arteriosclerosis, or a cause commonly unknown.

Sixth Nerve Palsy

The sixth nerve, the abducens nerve, has the longest intracranial course, and is most commonly affected by an intracranial injury such as blunt head trauma. It also can be involved in spontaneous partial paralysis of so-called ischemic cause (meaning cause unknown), more commonly with advancing age. Since the sixth nerve enervates the lateral rectus muscle, the one that pulls the eye toward the ear, partial or total paralysis results in the patient being cross-eyed. Diplopia is looking more to the side of the affected nerve and less, or perhaps not at all, to the other side. This results in a head turn to avoid double vision. Since diplopia is greater to one side, prisms in glasses are not so helpful. However, the temptation to cover or patch one eye should be avoided, if the head turn avoids diplopia. This is because spontaneous recovery is the greatest expectation, and patching one eye will delay recovery.

This is a situation also where physical therapy, like eye exercises, may take false credit for recovery, when spontaneous recovery is to expected anyway. Actually, the eye muscles controlling eye movement are 100 times stronger than needed for the job. However, coordination stimulated by nerve impulse is of primary importance in avoiding diplopia and promoting stereoptic vision. It probably would take months of total paralysis before the rectus muscles rotating the eye would show significant signs of atrophy (weakness). Surgery can be done, but obviously a long delay should occur before making this decision, due to high expectation of improvement in most cases.

Fourth Nerve Palsy

The fourth cranial nerve is called the trochlear nerve, and it innervates the superior oblique muscle. The superior oblique muscle may be affected by injury, especially if to the area of the orbit toward the nose, where the muscle is inserted. Acute ethmoid sinusitis in children can also cause palsy, which is probably more mechanical than due to nerve involvement. Then in older adults, spontaneous palsy of the superior oblique muscle can occur due to the fourth nerve palsy, and like the sixth nerve, it can have an "ischemic" type cause. In all cases, spontaneous recovery can be expected, especially in the ischemic variety. Diplopia and a head tilt are symptoms, but if fusion or binocular vision can be obtained by a head tilt, it is best not to patch or cover the eye. It most certainly would not be, as may be indicated by physical therapists, a good idea to cover the good eye in an attempt to "strengthen the weak eye." This is because the problem is not of a "weak muscle" but is actually a temporary neurological problem. Recovery is hastened by allowing the eyes to work together binocularly, especially if a head tilt is successful in avoiding diplopia. Since the double vision changes, depending on which way the eyes look, prisms in glasses are not helpful.

Third Nerve Palsy

The third cranial nerve is called the oculomotor nerve, and it enervates three muscles that move the eye, the elevating muscle of the upper eyelid, called the levator muscle, plus the pupil and the focusing muscles. Diabetes is one of the most common causes of spontaneous third nerve palsy, and cause unknown is still high on the list. A stroke can also cause third nerve palsy, as part of the more generalized stroke or as an isolated finding. Spontaneous recovery is again most likely. Diplopia is quite annoying, and the upper eyelid will droop (ptosis) until the complete third nerve palsy is resolved. In a way, drooping of the eyelid helps avoid double vision, and by the time the ptosis clears, the tendency for double vision has often also improved. If the pupil is not involved, then diabetes is the most likely cause (partial nerve palsy with pupillary sparing). A head turn or tilt is less likely to help avoid diplopia. If patching or occlusion of glasses is used, by all means do not cover the uninvolved eye. Forcing the involved eye to be used will not hasten recovery but will only make a person more miserable.

Some other causes of diplopia include thyroid eye disease and myasthenia gravis. Thyroid eye disease may be associated with exophthalmos and affect one eye more than the other. During the inflammatory phase the muscles swell, but may scar down later, with double vision mainly in upward gaze. Sometimes it is eventually necessary to release or recess the tightened inferior rectus surgically. Myasthenia is more likely to be associated with ptosis and with other systemic signs such as easy fatigability of the arms or legs.

Trigeminal Neuralgia (Tic Douloureux)

The trigeminal nerve, or the fifth cranial nerve, is a sensory nerve, involving the eye and facial tissues around the eye. It has three divisions: superior (ophthalmic), middle (maxillary), and lower (mandibular). It can be involved in neurological problems resulting from stoke, tumor, or injury, but the most common involvement is in regards what is called trigeminal neuralgia. Trigeminal neuralgia (tic douloureux) is a severe headache localized to the face, including the area around the eye. Treatment can involve surgery of the geniculate ganglion, which can relieve the pain, but may leave the eye numb, along with part of the face. Numbness of the eye can result in what would ordinarily be mild injury or infection, developing into a serious complication. The infraorbital branch serves the cheek, below the lower eyelid, and can be a factor in the diagnosis of orbital floor fracture when numbness is associated with trauma in the area. Numbness of the skin area below the eye, after a fist injury causing a black eye, for example, suggests that the floor of the orbit has been fractured, even before X-ray confirmation.

Bell's Palsy

Bell's palsy involves the seventh cranial nerve, also called the facial nerve. A spontaneous onset of Bell's palsy is usual, but the facial nerve may also be involved in a more generalized stroke. Because one side of the face is paralyzed, to varying degree, a person has trouble raising the eyebrow, blinking or closing the eye normally, or smiling due to sagging of the mouth, representing involvement of the three main branches of the facial nerve. Spontaneous improvement is to be expected with Bell's palsy, but it may take several months, and recovery may not be complete.

Initially, the most potential serious complication is related to not being able to close the eye for protection, especially during sleep. A special technique of closing the eye, with tape, at bedtime may be needed for awhile. If the problem is severe, or prolonged, it may be necessary to sew the eyelids together laterally, called tarsorrhaphy. This can be done in such a way that the eye can still see through the lid opening present toward the nose, and the closure can be reopened if recovery later occurs. Lubricants such as artificial tears and ointments can help protect the cornea from drying. Merely covering the eye with an eye patch or loose dressing may do more harm than good. Special taping techniques can be instructed by an eye doctor, as well as a way of helping to close the eye by traction on the outside corner (canthus) of the eyelids.

Recovery can be complicated by what is called aberrant regeneration of the facial nerve, meaning that regeneration can be misdirected. This can result in blinking or drooping of the upper eyelid when chewing or talking, or "crocodile" tears. Apparently a crocodile has tearing of the eyes when chewing, and aberrant regeneration of the seventh nerve in humans may cause the same sign, because the motor nerve to the lacrimal gland is also a function of the facial nerve.

Cerebral Vascular Accident (CVA)

CVA is a cerebral vascular accident, or a "stroke," and can cause double vision due to paralysis of the third (oculomotor), fourth (trochlear), fifth (facial), and sixth (abducens) nerves, or facial paralysis associated with the involvement of the seventh nerve. Such ocular nerve involvement may often be associated with paralysis of one side of the body and other problems. In such cases, as with prognosis for other cerebral deficits, there may or may not be recovery. In addition, there may be loss of a quarter or half of the side vision, either to the left or to the right, but affecting both eyes. This is called homonymous hemianopsia, or quadranopsia, depending on whether half or a quarter of the vision is involved in each eye. Sometimes, the loss of peripheral vision is the only neurological deficit, and then it is often called a "silent stroke." This is because, since there is no paralysis or other sign of stroke, the loss of side vision is sometimes not noticed initially. Spontaneous recovery can occur, but cannot be guaranteed. Physical therapists sometimes refer to the problem as "right-

or left-sided neglect," as if the peripheral vision problem can be improved by forced attention to that side. On the contrary, those with this problem should be allowed to have the TV, dinner, and conversation companions located on the side on which they see better, left or right, and not the other way around so as to exaggerate the problem. Credit for improvement, when it occurs, should not be falsely given to forcing one to pay attention to the "deficit." However, those with persistent homonymous hemianopsia should not be allowed to drive a car, even though they may adjust well to the problem by turning their head.

Myasthenia Gravis

Myasthenia gravis is a problem that also can manifest eye symptoms, sometimes as the initial problem. Drooping of the eyelid, or ptosis, often occurs, perhaps only when tired, initially. Also double vision can be intermittent as an early sign. These problems may worsen, especially with exercise, and become more permanent. Remissions occur and can be influenced by treatment. Diagnosis can be confirmed by Tensilon or ice testing. Placing ice over the affected muscles may eliminate double vision. Removal of the thymus gland often helps.

Headache

Headaches are a common reason to seek eye examination for logical reasons. There are different kinds of headaches, such as migraine, tension, sinus, cluster, and other neurological varieties. There is a natural concern that the need for glasses, or eye disease, can be a triggering cause for headaches. An eye exam can be useful to help in finding the cause of headaches, such as when there is evidence of papilledema, or swelling of the optic nerve, which can be caused by increased intracranial pressure. However, it is extremely uncommon that the need for glasses, or "eye strain," is a significant cause of headaches. Certainly, significant need for visual correction needs treatment. However, prolonged reading and the use of computers have spawned the idea that special treatments or eyeglasses are indicated, without scientific evidence that such uses of the eyes are harmful. Like other physical activity, it can be expected that expanded experience may result in "getting in shape," so that symptoms suggesting fatigue may diminish. In the meantime, such activities may be considered ocular gymnastics, which are not harmful to the eyes. Rest, and experience, will probably solve most such problems.

These are some special types of headaches:

1. Tension headaches are blamed on stress, and among the alleged causes may be prolonged computer use, incorrect posture, and sleep problems. These headaches can be frontal, above the eyes, or spread to the back of the neck. Episodes can be prolonged such that the cause needs to be investigated.
2. Sinus headaches cause pain around the eyes, above the eyes, or behind or below the eyes. Other symptoms such as those of a cold or sore throat may prolong the headache until the sinusitis clears.

3. Cluster headaches can be severe and very repetitive, localized around one eye. They may last for 30–60 minutes, recurring for weeks or months. Then they may spontaneously stop for months or years.

4. Migraine headaches are usually on one side of the head, moderate to severe, and often associated with nausea, enough to be called "sick headaches," whereby one tends to want to lay down. When a visual prodrome is involved, it is called classical migraine. Tingling or numbness of the hands or feet may occur. In women, hormones are often the trigger mechanism due to change, such as in premenstrual times.

5. Headaches due to eye problem problems will usually be accompanied by local signs of eye irritation, such as redness or discharge, foreign body sensation, sensitivity to light, drooping of the eyelid, or pain localized to the eyebrow. If the headache is due to an attack of angle closure glaucoma, there may be associated nausea and vomiting, redness of one eye with an enlarged pupil, and localization of the headache at the eyebrow.

Central Serous Retinopathy (Chorioretinopathy)

Central serous retinopathy (CSR) is a condition involving loss of vision to a variable degree, due to swelling of the macula. This syndrome mainly involves younger men, age twenty to forty-five, in one eye. Stereotypically, these men are hardworking and of the overachiever types, and the reasoning as to why an actual swelling of the macula is associated is not explainable. I was told that the treatment of this condition at the Mayo clinic was phenobarbital years ago.

The best news is that spontaneous recovery is expected without treatment, or change in life style, usually within three to four months. At one time laser treatment was offered to those in a hurry to get better, but it is now obvious that the best results come from doing nothing. Use of Diamox may hasten the decrease of swelling of the macula. Steroids are contraindicated since use of such can actually be a reason for developing such a problem, and even nose sprays.

Vision can completely return to normal, though there may be residual slight distorsion demonstrable on the amsler grid test, and a tiny yellow spot in the macula may persist. Occurrence in females are less common, and recurrences can happen.

15

HISTORY AND CURRENT DEVELOPMENTS IN REFRACTIVE SURGERY

REFRACTIVE SURGERY HISTORY

Refractive surgery has attracted tremendous interest and excitement, from its origin. Interest was so great, that marketing jumped ahead of scientific research, and though there have been great strides in new and better procedures, this is probably still true. As has been the case with many of the new surgical procedures, such as intraocular lens (IOL) implants, the innovators were those in private practice, not university programs where research projects may be expected to originate. Many of the original refractive surgeons were daring, innovative, and inventive, but were not necessarily held in high regard by their professional peers and were sometimes referred to as "cowboys." With time, and newer techniques, many more respected ophthalmic surgeons have become involved, and the approach to refractive surgery has become more conservatively acceptable.

Early refractive surgery marketing suggested that the procedure would become so common that every eye doctor, on every corner, would have a laser to do the job. In actuality, the technology has been so expensive and changing that only a few eye surgeons have "specialized" in refractive surgery. Even so, the number of refractive surgeons has not been insufficient for the demand, resulting in heavy price-cutting advertising. Such advertising tends to irritate the average ophthalmologist, for ethical reasons, and because the technique of refractive surgery does not approach the difficulty of most ophthalmic surgery, namely cataract surgery. One surgeon, experienced in both cataract and lasik surgery, rated the lasik surgery on a level of difficulty at as a three if rating the cataract surgery as a ten.

Another objection to advertising is the misleading impressions left with patients. One may get the impression that glasses will never be needed again, disregarding the imperfect result, and the natural process of presbyopia. Thus, a perfect distance result will not eliminate the need for reading glasses, an expected eventuality. Also, the uninformed may get the impression from advertisements that vision may become super and better than before: 20/20 or better. Of course, this refers to the improvement in uncorrected distance vision, without glasses, and does not reveal that vision can in no way become better than previously possible with correct glasses or contact lenses. On the other hand, due to "aberrations" resulting from lasik, the best corrected vision may actually be worse. Thus, though the uncorrected visual acuity may seem remarkably better, as from 20/400 to 20/30 for distance, the best corrected vision may have dropped from 20/20 to 20/30, though this is fortunately uncommon.

One of the manufacturers of refractive surgery materials has described the process as "vanity surgery." This well describes the goal: to reduce or eliminate the use of glasses. Like cosmetic plastic surgery, the procedure is not covered by health insurance. But like cosmetic plastic surgery, the rewards may be well worth the investment to a lot of people. A discussion of the options will follow. In spite of skeptics, the success of refractive surgery has become so common that the expectations of patients are increasingly difficult to satisfy. If the result is not absolutely perfect, the patients are inclined to ask for a repeat "enhancement" procedure.

The concept of refractive surgery is relatively new, in practice, if not in desire. Noting that scars of the cornea caused flattening, and/or astigmatism, experiments were performed, unfortunately usually on humans, in Japan and then Russia. As mentioned under "Anatomy of the Eye," the cornea, the curved window in front of the pupil is actually a greater factor in focusing light onto the retina than the lens of the eye. The cornea cannot change its shape to allow better focusing, like the lens can, but the shape of the cornea can be altered. Nearsighted eyes are larger than average or have a cornea more curved than average or a combination of both. We cannot shrink the eye, but we can flatten the cornea, an idea that spawned the idea of refractive surgery. Initially this was with "radial keratotomy" and then laser treatments.

Radial keratotomy was probably the original refractive surgery procedure (that is if you exclude the introduction of intraocular lenses in cataract surgery). This technique involves making deep incisions, like cutting segments of a pie, in four to eight incisions radiating from a central 4–6 mm zone of clear cornea, depending on the needed result for correcting the degree of myopia. Horizontal incisions in the midperiphery were used to correct astigmatism. By modern standards, this radial keratotomy surgery was pretty much "by guess and by gosh," but the early results were often quite exciting for nearsighted people. Unfortunately, early modifications to achieve even more perfect results were often performed, often too early, before the long-term results showed that actually too much had been performed initially. Premature enthusiasm for results too often ended in later lament for what is called "hyperopic shift," meaning the cornea flattened even more with time. Having switched from being nearsighted to being farsighted, this often resulted in premature reading problems and eventually poor vision at all distances, without glasses. Improvements resulted from experience such that the results could be better controlled. However, newer and better refractive procedures developed, so that, to my knowledge, radial keratotomy is no longer performed. Another long-term complication is the adverse effect of radial keratotomy on the evaluation of intraocular implant calculations if cataract surgery becomes necessary. It is interesting that those who have had radial keratotomy are not so critical of their surgeons, as if they better understand that they were taking a chance, and it just didn't work out.

Following radial keratotomy came the laser procedures. As mentioned, flattening of the cornea reduces myopia (nearsightedness). Flattening the surface with a laser, as with photorefractive keratectomy (PRK), involves destroying the epithelium, making the eye painful for days until the epithelium can regrow. When lasik developed, it meant avoiding the pain by making a flap of the cornea, beneath the surface epithelium, and then applying the laser treatment to deeper corneal tissue. The flap then is allowed to fall back in place and seal itself without sutures. The procedure is so amazingly painless, and the result so good instantly, that the routine has become to do both eyes together. To overcome hyperopia (farsightedness) it is desirable to increase the roundness of the cornea, something not possible with radial keratotomy, and more difficult, but possible, with lasik. Astigmatism also can be corrected. Further new developments include the ability to create the corneal flap with the laser also, making the surgical part of the use of metallic cutting instruments unnecessary. Other advancements include improved lasers and measuring devices so that results can be more predictable. "Wave Front technology claims to be able to improve on visual aberrations such that vision is actually improved, over preoperative abilities, and even if not likely to be true, should at least improve the results of refractive surgery.

TYPES OF REFRACTIVE SURGERY

PRK (Photo Refractive Keratectomy)

Now some refer to this as advanced surface ablation (ASA). This is the original laser surgery for reshaping the cornea. Technology allows changing the shape of the cornea with laser, to flatten centrally to correct nearsightedness and alter the shape to correct astigmatism. The results are predictable, but the early stages are complicated by pain. Removal of the epithelial surface of the eye creates one massively "scratched cornea," and since the cornea is extremely sensitive, the eye is so painful that only one eye is usually treated at a time. The epithelial cover regrows such that the function of the eye is not altered. The newest methods of pain relief and the use of therapeutic contact lenses have rejuvenated interest in this original laser procedure. It is estimated that ophthalmic surgeons are now doing about 20–30 percent PRK now. The military prefers this type treatment for their pilots, for safety reasons. Radial keratotomy, for example, was not allowed for the police or military due to the fact that it weakened the eye in cases of injury, such as a blow to the eye. PRK is recommended for thinner corneas, rather than lasik. Indications: = mild or moderate degrees of myopia and astigmatism.

Lasik

Laser in situ keratomileusis (Lasik) has led to the most rapid increase in interest in refractive surgery. It has accounted for the highest volume of refractive surgery. The immediate impact of Lasik is due to the fact that it is relatively painless, and both eyes can be done initially. The lack of pain is due to the fact that the epithelial surface covering is not scraped away. A thin flap of superficial cornea is lifted surgically (or, more recently, by laser), the laser treatment applied to the bed of the cornea exposed, and the flap repositioned. It takes about 10 minutes per eye, and the visual improvement is relatively instant. Long-term results have been good, without the complications experienced with radial keratotomy. Complications can occur, including infection and problems with the flap of corneal tissue, but are not common. Halos around lights can occur with those with large pupils. Innovations in technology have made results more predictable and more perfect. Indications are for mild or moderate degrees of myopia (nearsightedness). Farsightedness and astigmatism can also be treated, to a somewhat lesser degree.

Limitations involve extreme myopia, thin corneas, and large pupils. Some refractive surgeons regret the way lasik was pushed beyond safe limits in trying to correct high degrees of myopia, in the early stages of use rather than await long-term results. A new innovation called Intralase utilizes "all laser,"

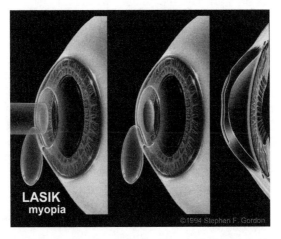

This illustration shows a flap of cornea laid back, with laser applied to the deeper stromal bed. Then it shows the cornea is relatively flatter once the flap is put back in place. Please understand that the illustration is made to exaggerate what happens, the amounts of tissue being more microscopic in actual practice. Copyright © 1994 Stephen F. Gordon.

meaning a laser is used to fashion the flap, rather than a steel microkeratome. In addition to more accuracy, it may be possible to work on thinner corneas. Other innovative advances include technology allowing greater accuracy if a patient does not hold completely still, or if corneal aberrations are present. In spite of all these improvements, the incidence of lasik surgery reportedly has flattened since 2001, contrary to an expected increased interest.

Laser-Assisted Subepithelial Keratectomy (Lasek) or Epi-Lasik

This newer variation of Lasik involves a thinner flap including just epithelium. Therefore the pain factor is still present to a degree, but corneal thickness is less of a problem. In Lasek, the epithelium is removed in a sheet, after treatment with alcohol. With Epi-lasik, the epithelial flap is raised by a special keratome-like instrument. Along with PRK, the eventual results visually may actually improve on Lasik results, but overall indications are about the same, with a thin cornea and large pupils being less of a contraindication. Some argue that this is not a significant improvement over PRK in the long term.

Intrastromal Corneal Ring (Intac)

The main advantage of this procedure is that it is reversible. A thin ring of plastic material is placed in the superficial corneal subepithelial tissue, which flattens the central cornea. It works mainly on lower degrees of myopia. The ring can be removed, restoring the original corneal shape. Another indication can be keratoconus, a corneal disease involving increased central curvature. This is not a preferred procedure by most refractive surgeons.

Conductive Keratoplasty (CK)

This procedure is designed to appeal to the presbyopic group, those emmetropic for distance, and especially those hyperopic for distance. It is FDA approved in monovision form, meaning that one eye is for reading and the other for distance vision. Instead of laser, radio frequency energy is used in a circular pattern on the midperiphery of the cornea, creating puncturelike burns. This heat reaction causes a central puckering, or steepening, so as to become rounder, thus becoming relatively myopic (less hyperopic). No scars result, and in fact the results are not expected to be permanent. Retreatment is possible. The monovision idea can be used as in other forms of refractive surgery, but it is useful to know in advance if a person will tolerate monovision. The results can be simulated by trial of contact lenses preoperatively. The results may be quite satisfactory but cannot be expected to be as good visually as with glasses, especially with increasing age. If the "better eye" meant for distance is 0.75 diopters or up to 3 diopters farsighted, then both eyes can be treated. As in monovision with contact lenses, there is a limit to acceptable binocularity, meaning that the "reading eye" probably would not give satisfactory vision for all needs beyond the age of mid to late fifties. The recent trend toward "light-touch" techniques has given better and even more lasting effects.

Phakic IOLs

This is an invasive surgical procedure in which an intraocular lens is inserted into the eye, either in front or behind the pupil, but leaving the normal lens of the eye in place. It is indicated for more extreme degrees of myopia (nearsightedness), for example, 12 to 20 diopters, or for extreme hyperopia (farsightedness). Limiting factors include the cost of intraocular surgery, and potential complications, such as cataract, infection, or any of the rare complications involving intraocular surgery, including possible loss of the eye. The IOL can be removed, for exchange, or when cataract surgery becomes necessary. A corneal test called an endothelial cell count can be done preoperatively to measure the health of the cornea and give an idea of how any further intraocular surgery may be tolerated.

Accommodative IOLs

This approach represents the newest, the most extreme, and perhaps the procedure with the greatest future in refractive surgery. What is new is that intraocular lens implants are designed to change focus such that an operated eye may be expected to see both for distance, and closer, with changes of accommodation somewhat like the focusing ability of an eye before presbyopia occurs. Standard cataract surgery resulting in aphakia always leaves the eye in a state of relative fixed focus; in other words, glasses are required to perfect distance and close vision: aphakik bifocal spectacles. When intraocular lenses were devised, the eye was also left in relative fixed focus. If perfect for distance, the eye needed help for close vision. This, however, was probably similar to the situation before surgery, if the cataract patient was of the usual senior stage of age.

Pseudo-accommodative IOLs

These are implants that are multifocal, like a bifocal, but usually involving concentric areas of different refraction. The Array lens has been in use, and new lenses, such as the ReStor and ReZoom lenses, are big improvements. The design of these lenses is similar to that tried with contact lenses, which were not very successful.

Intracorneal Inlay

This is a procedure not yet FDA approved, involving the creation of a lamellar corneal flap followed by the insertion of an inlay lens, centered over the pupil. It is being offered to hyperopes or myopes, but not recommended with much astigmatism, or too flat or thin corneas. If approved, it has the advantage that it may be done in the doctor's office, and may also be performed with an aspheric inlay, which provides another solution to presbyopia by offering near-vision correction as well. Supposedly the inlay may be replaced or removed, but potential hazards of the procedure make some skeptical.

Multifocal Lasik

This is being done experimentally, and theoretically offers the same advantages as pseudoaccommodative IOLs. Limitations will be in regard to dissatisfaction with results visually, plus the expected halos and reduced contrast problems in vision. Also, there is the question of reversibility of the procedure.

What should you do? Which procedure should you have done? Well, I believe you should be given options, and your primary eye doctor should help you decide. For most people, the option of wearing glasses, as needed, is probably still the best. A refractive surgeon has said that if a person is used to good vision with glasses, bifocals, or trifocals, that they should probably not have the accommodative IOL instead of the conventional IOL at the time of cataract surgery, because they may not be satisfied with the visual result.

Those wearing contact lenses have the option of monovision when they become presbyopic, and this gives them opportunity to decide if they may want monovision options with later refractive surgery, or cataract surgery. Those who are mildly nearsighted should probably not even consider refractive surgery. To be able to read without glasses at a reasonable distance is something to be cherished in later years, and young people need to be told this *with emphasis*: What I mean by this is, those less than 3 diopters nearsighted. This is among the highest of postoperative complaints among myopes: that one cannot see as well up close anymore even though this was mentioned in the preoperative exam.

As far as timing is concerned, it is a matter of not too early and not too late. A young person may make the mistake of having lasik too early, before their eyes have stopped changing, and then become more nearsighted later. Most people have reached this stage by the mid twenties. However, if a young person waits too long, then the period of "perfect vision" is shortened, before presbyopia sets in.

Among the experts, some guidelines have been set. From -1 to -8 diopters nearsightedness, a form of Lasik is preferred. From -8 to -12 diopters, it is about equal between Lasik and phakic IOLs, and from -12 to -20 diopters, phakic IOLs are recommended for such high degrees of nearsightedness (myopia). For farsightedness, the ranges vary. The results of lasik are limited for farsightedness, probably to less than 3 diopters. CK can be good, and the fact that the results are often not permanent may be an advantage, both for enhancements, or and for further developments such as cataract surgery. For higher degrees of farsightedness (hyperopia) phakic IOLs or accommodative IOLs would be necessary.

What are the downsides, or the complications? Cost is one potential problem, and though people do not want to spend any more for a procedure than necessary, we are also the best to remember the old statement about getting what we pay for. The surgeon to whom I refer charges from $4,000 to $5,000 for bilateral procedures such as Lasik and CK. Phakic IOLs (intraocular lens implants) are roughly double in cost. Remember, insurance is not likely to be of any help. The biggest complication is probably not being quite satisfied with the result. The most common complaints center around not being perfect for distance, and then as mentioned, there are those nearsighted who just did not quite understand that they will no longer see up close as well as they did before surgery. Distance imperfections can be improved by touchup enhancement procedures in Lasik, once or even twice. However, to undo a lasik procedure so as to see better for close is not practical. Halos around lights, at least temporarily, are a common complaint following Lasik, especially if one has large pupils normally, and this is why pupil measurement is important preoperatively. Phakic IOLs can be replaced, but cataract and corneal complications may occur, things already of concern following the primary procedure. Trying to replace an accommodative IOL would be even riskier. Revision agreements should be revealed preoperatively.

I recently received a promotion announcement from a refractive surgeon describing a new phakic IOL, a lens inserted in front of the normal lens for nearsighted people. A fee of $4,500 per eye was quoted, including outpatient facilities and anesthesia, cost of the lens, postoperative lasik enhancement if necessary (like for astigmatism), and $500 stipend for the patient's comanagement, should this be elected. This shows how such agreements are presented.

PRESBYOPIA SURGERY

Presbyopia is defined as age related loss of focusing ability to see up close, near vision. Onset is gradual, and the emmetrope, one whose eyes are naturally in focus without focusing at a distance, notes beginning problems by the mid-forties, and progressively with increased age.

The cause of presbyopia is debated, but most agree the problem is a result of the aging process of the normal lens of the eye. Hardening or sclerosis of the lens material, not weakness of the eye muscles, makes it relatively progressively unresponsive to efforts of focusing muscles of the eye.

How can presbyopia be prevented? Well, don't get any older, heh heh. Recently claims have been made that antioxidants in leafy vegetables may help, and there is a study being performed utilizing eye drops containing antioxidants. Also dark sunglasses have been proposed, suggesting that sun exposure is a cause. However, no diet, exercise, medicine, or modification of life style has been scientifically proven to be helpful.

Management or treatment of the problem is usually in the form of proper spectacles, or eye glasses of sufficient focusing power to satisfy one's best visual potential. Some go to the drug store and try out what is available until they feel they have solved the problem. Others just ignore the problem and limit visual activity. And some are even willing to try surgical means to avoid glasses. Several options are actually available, such as contact lenses and laser procedures. These include monovision or bifocal contact lenses, laser treatments of the cornea to create monovision or multifocal solutions, radio wave corneal treatment called CK, and now also the intraocular surgical approach.

The surgical management of presbyopia is the newest approach attracting attention directed to the consumer. The earliest surgery was directed to the ciliary body, the tissue behind the iris, the colored part of the eye, which gives support to the lens of the eye. Wedge inserts into the ciliary body have been tried, but results have not been encouraging. More recently, surgery has been directed to removing the lens of the eye and replacing it with a special artificial lens in an attempt to restore the function of a younger, natural lens. Yes, this can mean doing a cataract operation, even if you do not have a cataract, which is called clear lens extraction. It is not so extreme, of course, if you do have a cataract, and accommodative IOLs have been approved by the FDA as an alternative for those who need cataract surgery. The result is then called pseudophakik presbyopia correction (PPC), as compared to pseudophakia, the term applied to the condition of the eye after conventional IOL surgery.

Results have been good enough such that interest is developing among those who want to avoid glasses as much as possible. Conventional intraocular implants used in cataract surgery can be selected to offer good distance vision, often such that distance glasses are no longer needed. However, the conventional IOL is not multifocal, so reading glasses are required. If dealing with cataract patients, it is quite appealing to be able to see after surgery, without glasses, though it is true that most cataract patients are old enough that they have already learned to live with glasses. Refractive surgery patients who are interested in getting rid of thick distance glasses must deal with the fact that glasses would be eventually needed for reading, once they becomes presbyopic. They thus might feel that their glasses-free goal would be compromised. The lure of being able to see at all distances, without glasses, may attract such refractive surgery patients to presbyopia surgery.

The largest group potentially eligible for presbyopia surgery would be the emmetropes, 40 percent of the total population, who naturally see just fine until their arms get too short in their forties. The emmetropic group is estimated as 55 million in the United States, 44 million of whom are naturally that way, and others achieving this, following refractive or cataract surgery. Those marketing ways of avoiding glasses are naturally attracted to this large group of potential clients.

Treatment of presbyopia can be approached in different ways. As mentioned, refractive surgery usually involves changing the curvature of the cornea, the clear window tissue in front of the pupil. This is usually done with a laser these days, but there is a new technique of inserting a wafer-thin reading lens into the center of the cornea. The biggest new trend though involves removing the natural lens, behind the pupil, and replacing it either with an IOL, which moves so as to simulate the focusing ability of the normal lens (thus showing that the focusing muscles still work), or with a multifocal lens. Multifocal lenses are not all one power. For example, the central part may be for close vision and the peripheral part for distance vision. Multifocal IOLs are therefore not true accommodative lenses, but are pseudoaccommodative in their action.

Market analysis has predicted many people to be interested in presbyopic surgery. Cost, of course, is a limiting factor. A high percentage of people having had intraocular presbyopia surgery, perhaps 80–90 percent, say they can function without glasses most of the time. Patient selection is, of course, important if expecting good results. It has been said, however, that those patients who have been wearing glasses most of the time, of a multifocal nature, such as bifocals or trifocals, *may not be satisfied with the visual result of presbyopia surgery.* However, people who have been avoiding glasses by use of contact lenses, or plain neglect, will probably be most satisfied. Also, those for whom cost is not a deterrent, and who have been avoiding glasses, may be good candidates.

As far as cost is concerned, of course insurance does not cover presbyopia surgery, much the same as cosmetic surgery. What is a big surprise, however, is that Medicare has agreed to allow a form of balance billing for cataract surgery, something it never allowed before. Surgeons are allowed to bill Medicare for the cataract surgery, and they will pay their usual fee. The surgeons are also allowed to then bill the patients for "presbyopia surgery" (a term I personally have a problem with), which allows the surgeons to collect directly from the patients the extra cost of the special intraocular implant and the additional surgical fee. Secondary insurance, following the lead of Medicare as usual, would be expected to pay the usual amount it pays for cataract surgery, but not for the additional presbyopia surgery.

The additional amount charged the patient may vary, but is around $2,800 per eye (a range of quotations from $1,100 to $3,200). This may seem like not so bad a deal for those who go to the extreme to avoid glasses, at any cost, but not such a good deal for the elderly cataract patient who is used to Medicare covering everything. It is expected that most elderly patients will continue to have conventional intraocular lens implants, because they want Medicare to pay for everything.

Presbyopia Surgery Alternatives

Monovision Lasik

This is the most common and the most proven approach to providing both distance and near vision. Certainly, experience with contact lenses has shown this to be quite successful, and frankly more successful than attempts at bifocal and other multifocal contact lenses. It works well with myopes from −1 to −8, hyperopes from +2.5 to +3, and those with less than 3 diopters of astigmatism. It is not recommended for athletes, pilots, or truck drivers, or anyone who insists on not having to wear glasses at any time for anything. Patients can be told that the monovision can be reversed if they prefer binocularity for distance, but it is preferable to have tested the acceptance of monovision preoperatively. Even so, it has been noted that people tend to be more critical and demanding of perfection after surgery.

Accommodative IOL (Lens Extraction)

As mentioned, this involves removing the normal lens of the eye and replacing it with an IOL, the difference being that the lens inserted has the ability to change shape in a way to simulate normal focusing or accommodation. The most well known of such a lens is the Crystalens (Eyeonics). Others lenses are being used, and more are in the experimental stages, such as being able to replace the gel-like normal lens material with a synthetic gel also able to change shape as does the normal youthful lens of the eye. Other new accommodative IOLs are in the wings such as the Safarazi (B&L) and Smart IOL (Medennium), and more are coming in such as the Synchrony Dual Optic IOL (Visiogen), the Kellan TetraFlex (Lenstec), the NuLens (Herzeliya, Israel), and the light Adjustable IOL (Calhoun Vision).

Multifocal IOL (Lens Extraction)

There are many such lenses, including the ReStor (Alcon), Array (AMO), ReZoom (AMO), and Tecnis (AMO). Some such lenses are better for close vision (Restor) than others; some are better for intermediate visual needs (Rezoom). For these reasons, some surgeons suggest a combination of one type of lens in one eye, and another in the second eye. Complications include difficulty in adjusting to multifocal images, glare, halos, and diminished clarity of vision. These complications have shown a lessening degree of problems with newer multifocal lenses.

Phakic Multifocal IOL

This involves insertion of an intraocular implant in front of the normal lens of the eye, as can be done for high degrees of hyperopia or myopia but also available for lower degrees of hyperopia or myopia, so as to be able to also provide the ability to see up close. The downside includes the fact that this is an intraocular surgical procedure, with similar potential complications and increased cost. Also, there is the expectation of causing a cataract, though only reported in 4 percent, and thus requiring another operation later.

Scleral Surgery

This is a lesser-known but different approach to solving the problems of presbyopia. Advantages include not having to disturb the clear cornea or perform intraocular surgery.

a. Anterior Ciliary Sclerotomy—this procedure spun off the notation that if radial keratotomy incisions were carried across the limbus, the junction of the cornea with the adjacent sclera (thereby over the ciliary body tissue), that presbyopia symptoms were less noticeable. Such incisions, when made to help reduce presbyopia symptoms, have sometimes been complicated by anterior segment ischemia (poor blood supply to the area), or more commonly by poor visual results.

b. Laser presbyopia reversal (LAPR) utilizes infrared laser tissue ablation to create radial incisions that remove a groove of scleral tissue overlying the ciliary body. This has been approved in Europe but not yet in the United States.

c. Scleral Expansion Bands (SEB) procedure, also known as the Scleral Spacing Procedure (SSP), involves creating radial anterior ciliary body incisions and a scleral tunnel between pairs of incisions, and placing an implant into one of the scleral tunnels. Complications include ineffectiveness and scleral prolapse (herniation of deeper tissues).

Conductive Keratoplasty (CK)

For this procedure radio frequency energy is applied to the corneal stroma (intermediate layer) by means of a probe tip inserted into the peripheral cornea at 8 to 32 treatment points to produce a contracting effect that increases the curvature of the central cornea. It is best to treat +1.5 diopters or less hyperopia for a long term of greater than one year, as long as there is minimal astigmatism.

The procedure is considered very safe but not as effective or accurate as lasik, and it takes more time. Complications include transient astigmatism and temporary effect, resulting in the need to retreat in one year, or select another procedure. However, the latest results with "light touch" have been a bit more encouraging regards duration. It is considered less important in the future of refractive surgery and of "uncertain advantage."

Multifocal Lasik

In this presbyopic lasik procedure the ablation profile has been modified to create an aspheric curvature of the corneal bed so as to create better near vision, along with good distance vision. Patients need be informed that distance vision will be temporarily blurred, while near vision will be immediately good. Utilizing some monovision helps long-term result, and enhancement is available two to three years later. "Presby-Lasik" patients of hyperopic type, plus those who are pseudophakik (already had cataract surgery), are among the most pleased post treatment. Problems include the fact that there may develop a loss of best-corrected vision, one or two lines on the Snellen chart, and the duration of positive effect lasts five to seven years.

Intracorneal Inlay

An aspheric inlay is placed under a lamellar flap of the cornea and centered over the pupil, such as the ReVision IOL, best for hyperopes, 1–6 diopters, with low astigmatism. It is "more lasting" than CK, but not yet FDA approved.

So who should have presbyopia surgery? Currently, the biggest market is for those with cataracts and those who can afford the extra cost, perhaps 25–30 percent of those with cataracts. The big potential market is among those who do not have cataracts but want to see without glasses. If you are someone who requires strong eyeglasses, you may be better motivated. Then there are those who have been avoiding glasses and now can see that they are going to need glasses, but are willing to go to great expense to continue to avoid glasses. Such people are targeted by the presbyopic surgery industry.

The movable part implant gives variable focus, like the original lens, but to a limited degree, such that it may not be satisfactory for very small print or things held very close. One multifocal lens is good for distance and for small print but not so good at intermediate distances, like for a computer. Another multifocal lens gives good intermediate vision, but is not so good for small print up closer.

When discussing the effects of different intraocular lenses, Dr. Wm. W. Maloney reports in *Ocular Surgical News*, the May 1, 2006, issue, that there are five zones of focus to consider. Zone 1 is for near-vision ability to see newsprint and sewing; Zone 2 is for things such as computers or menus; Zone 3 is for indoor TV, cooking, and eating; Zone 4 is for daytime driving, golf, or tennis; and Zone 5 is for nighttime driving, movies, and theater. None of the available presbyopia correcting IOLs can deliver good vision in all five zones. These IOLs currently include four alternatives: Crystalens (Eyeonics), ReZoom (Advanced Medical Optics), ReStor (Alcon), and conventional IOLs. To achieve the desired effects for close work, a form of binocular "blending" is suggested, making one or both eyes a bit nearsighted, especially if Zone 5 night-driving requirements are not so important, and could be solved with a rarely needed pair of driving glasses.

Under the circumstances, some suggest using one type of lens in one eye and another in the second eye to take advantage of the best of each lens. However, most surgeons believe that it is best to use the same lens in both eyes and suggest a short interval between doing the eyes, such as three weeks. Why do both eyes with multifocal lenses, with a short interval between surgeries? One reason is that it is necessary for the brain to adjust to the multiple images in order to select the correct image, and it is probably easier if both eyes have the same needs (problems). How does it do this? It reminds me of the story about three guys arguing about the most important invention in the world. One said the airplane, another said the spacecraft, and the third said the thermos. Why the thermos, he was asked, and he said "Well, when you put something cold in it, it stays cold, and when you put something hot it, it stays hot." When queried as to what was so special about that, he replied, "Well, how do it know?" With multifocal lenses, the brain needs to "know," and apparently it "do," demonstrating tremendous ability of the brain to adjust.

What if the brain does not adapt? Symptoms of dysphotopsia are described with multifocal lenses, including reflections, temporal darkness or visual field defect, unsettling vision arc, glare, and central flash and halos. The solution, is usually waiting for the symptoms to go away per "neural adaptation," which may take nine months or more. But if a patient cannot tolerate the symptoms, the multifocal lens can be replaced with an accommodative IOL, such as Crystalens, or by a conventional monofocal implant. Dr. Maloney states in *Ocular News*, October 1, 2006, issue, that pseudophakia monovision is different than contact lens monovision, and it takes the brain only one or two days to adjust, even without preoperative testing.

Complications of intraocular presbyopia surgery can include anything that can go wrong with intraocular surgery, including infection, retinal detachment, macular swelling, corneal decompensation, and other causes of loss of vision. With routine cataract surgery, these complications are now fortunately rare, and the same might be expected for presbyopia surgery. The biggest complications would be failure to achieve the visual results expected, but this can be lessened by patient selection and education. An unknown for the younger patient, in their forties or fifties, is if later in life they may develop macular degeneration and be handicapped by having a multifocal IOL which makes the symptoms worse, or if glaucoma will develop and difficulty in evaluating the visual field tests will result from having a multifocal IOL in place. Also, those who have had Lasik may find that additional aberrations created by the multifocal lens may be more intolerable.

So presbyopia surgery is not without reason for concern, as should be observed with any surgery. It is true that an unsatisfactory result can be corrected by removal and replacement of the intraocular implant. However, this can be more difficult than the original surgery, and the complication rate increases. It is best to carefully select patients as to their expectations, give them detailed preoperative information, and then avoid reoperations if possible. It is not like returning a shirt to Nordstroms to get one that fits better.

Where should you go to get presbyopic surgery? Not all cataract surgeons perform presbyopic surgery. Some ophthalmic surgeons currently decline because of skepticism about indications and/or expected results, or difficulty answering the question from a patient as to whether they would have the surgery themselves. Though any good cataract surgeon can probably do presbyopic surgery, some lens manufacturers require that an ophthalmologist must take their special training course and be certified by them before they will allow the ophthalmic surgeon to buy their lens.

Many refractive surgeons advertise, something doctors did not use to do prior to deregulation in the 1970s, but which has become more common in competition with other high-volume surgeons. High-volume surgeons are also likely to encourage and attract referrals. This brings up the subject of comanagement, meaning that the referring doctor, quite often an optometrist, assumes the postoperative care, with approval and support of the surgeon. As mentioned, this is an automatic routine with lasik-type refractive surgery, but the ability of an optometrist to assume postoperative cataract care has been a source of dispute between ophthalmology and optometry leadership groups. Another related issue is that, since Medicare is involved in paying fees, which include a follow-up of about ninety days, it needs to be established preoperatively as to what fees the patient may be expected to be charged postoperatively, say by the referring doctor, relative to the follow-up of the presbyopia surgical part of the procedure.

Presbyopia surgery is certainly new and exciting. Dr. Wm. W. M. Maloney describes presbyopia correction as the most important innovation in ophthalmic surgery since phacoemulsification (small-incision cataract surgery). Since there was an increase in the use of phacoemulsification, from 9 percent to 95 percent between 1985 and 1995, there may also be a marked increase of usage of this newest innovative procedure in the future. Though there are reasons for concern and skepticism, the idea has obvious merit, and newer better implants are in the works. So waiting awhile before deciding about having this surgery is not a bad idea. However, if grandma comes home after cataract surgery and can see better without glasses than anyone else in the family, some jealousy may stimulate action.

16

SOME UNUSUAL EYE PROBLEMS AND EYE INJURIES

EYE PROBLEMS

Cancer of the Eye

Fortunately cancer does not often affect the eye. Primary cancers include retinoblastoma (occurs in children at an early age), ocular melanomas, and eyelid tumors.

Retinoblastoma may be present at birth but usually is not diagnosed until eighteen to twenty-four months of age. It is one of the most common childhood malignancies and fortunately rare, sometimes familial. Diagnosis is too often delayed until the child's pupil is noted to be white or the eye turns outward. It can be bilateral, and treatment of choice is enucleation (removal of the eye), which can be curative if performed early enough. Newer treatments may preserve vision and life.

Melanomas of the eye are the most common primary malignant tumors of the eyeball. The usual site is in the "choroid," the pigment containing vascular layer beneath the retina, in the back of the eye. Diagnosis is usually a result of eye examination, and of course diagnostic biopsy is difficult, but now not impossible. A biopsy specimen can be obtained via a 25-gauge needle, and new genetic typing procedure can predict the likelihood of metastasis. Treatment has usually been enucleation, but other localized radiation treatments are being performed. Clinically there are signs that may help differentiate a malignant melanoma from a benign melanoma (nevus). Metastasis, or spread of the tumor elsewhere in the body, may lead to death, like with other melanomas.

Iris melanomas are less common, and since there is a differential diagnosis of benign melanoma, observation may be initially the course of management. Eyelid melanomas are quite rare, and conjunctival melanomas can also occur. Biopsy of the conjunctiva or the eyelid is possible so as to differentiate benign nevi, which are quite common, from malignant tumors.

Basal cell carcinomas and squamous cell carcinomas occur on the eyelids. They can be locally excised.

The most common metastatic tumor to of the eye is from breast cancer to the choroid, and this is quite unusual.

Corneal Dystrophy

The anatomy of the cornea has been described as very unique. Remaining perfectly clear, like a window, it also is unique in that it has no blood vessels to provide nourishment. On the outside, the corneal epithelium and a special layer called Bruch's membrane provide protection. On the inside, a special layer of cells called the endothelium helps keep the cornea from becoming swollen by fluids bathing the interior, and yet also selectively allows penetration of needed nutrients from these fluids called aqueous.

With age, the number of healthy endothelial cells diminishes naturally. This means that any trauma or surgery affecting this tissue, including cataract surgery, is less well tolerated. Invasive surgery, such as cataract surgery, causes the endothelial cell count to go down further. If the endothelial cell count becomes too low, then the protective ability of the endothelium to keep fluid out of the cornea diminishes, and the cornea becomes swollen and less clear.

There is a condition called endothelial corneal dystrophy, which can spontaneously reduce the endothelial health dramatically. As a result, typical spots, called guttata, can be seen with microscopic examination, leading to diagnosis of a condition called Fuch's endothelial dystrophy, a condition predominating in women and often familial.

In the earliest stages, the diagnosis is one mainly of potential, if guttata are evident. However, with time, evidence of corneal swelling results, which causes blurring of vision. Typically, this is, in the early stages, early in the day. This is because the normal activity of wakeful hours results in evaporation-type reduction of fluid from the windowlike cornea. Eventually, the swelling can be identified by reduced vision and microscopic examination evidence of swelling of the cornea. The swelling of the cornea can be accurately measured by a special instrument called a pachymeter, which measures the thickness of the cornea. Treatment can involve use of hypertonic solutions or ointments to draw water out of the cornea, allowing better vision. Later stages of corneal swelling results in fluid extending to the surface of the eye, causing blisters, or bullae, and this is called bullous keratopathy. When one of these bullae ruptures to allow drainage of the waterlike fluid, pain results similar to any corneal abrasion. However, since the cornea is not healthy, healing usually takes longer. Such worsening may lead to a need for a corneal transplant operation, but it is not inevitable that all patients reach this stage.

A corneal transplant amounts to replacing the central portions of the cornea with a donor cornea, from someone who recently died and whose corneas were donated. This full thickness graft therefore caries with it a healthier endothelium. It is not necessary to match blood cell types between donor and recipient. The results can be quite good, when considering restoration of vision, but survival of the graft is not guaranteed, and a repeat procedure may be required. Astigmatism of significant degree often complicates vision correction.

There are several more rare types of corneal dystrophy, most of which do not significantly affect vision, and represent various types of opacities of the cornea, which may not be evident without microscopic (slit lamp) examination.

A very common corneal variation, like a dystrophy, is the grey ring that forms around the peripheral cornea, making the eye color less distinctive. This condition is called, arcus: arcus senilis for the older people, and arcus juvenilis for the younger people. The grey-colored material is mainly cholesterol, and may represent a high level of serum cholesterol, but most of the time, it is not related to high cholesterol levels. Nevertheless, it can be quite noticeable, especially in brown-eyed people, and these people need to be assured that it is not threatening to vision because it is limited to the peripheral cornea where it does not obstruct the visual axis. Often it is hereditary.

Chorioretinitis

The choroid is a layer of tissue beneath the retina, containing blood vessels and pigment, and is the most posterior part of the uveal layer, being contiguous with the iris in front, and the ciliary body in the middle of the eye. Blood-borne diseases can affect this layer, causing visual problems sometimes, or forming scars, which can suggest that some form of chorioretinitis (inflammation of the choroid and adjacent retina) was present, when discovered in the course of fundus eye examination, usually as part of a routine examination.

Histoplasmosis is a flulike illness due to a soil fungus most common in the Midwest part of this country. In most cases, signs of how this involved the eye are present in the form of tiny round scars in the retina, and sometimes a halo of mild scarring around the optic nerve. Finding these signs suggests POH, or presumed ocular histoplasmosis. Sometimes, however, there can be neo-vascular membrane (new blood vessels) formation in the macular region, and bleeding from these vessels can cause wet-type macular degeneration, even in a younger person. Diagnosis can be confirmed by flourescein angiography, and treatment can be attempted as performed with the wet form of age-related macular degeneration.

Toxoplasmosis is another flulike illness, which can leave its mark on the eyes. It is caused by parasitic organisms carried by animals, such as cats. Little cysts spread around the body, including the eyes, and these may remain dormant for years. Rupture of these cysts may cause symptoms of inflammation from floaters in vision to actual reduction of vision, especially if the macula, the sensitive reading vision part of the eye, is involved. Most serious is the congenital form, whereas wherein the infection is transmitted during pregnancy to the fetus, and the eye involvement may be severe. The mother, however, would not transmit this problem to subsequent eventual pregnancies. Treatment with medication is available, but there can be side effects.

Retinitis Pigmentosa

This problem, sometimes called RP, is a disease primarily involving the rods of the retina, the peripheral retinal cells needed for night vision. It is almost always hereditary, with the onset of symptoms of night blindness beginning in the first and second decades of life. Driving a car at night eventually becomes hazardous. Though vision may continue to be 20/20 for some time, typical pigmentation of the retina of "bone corpuscular" nature tips off the problem during eye examination. A visual field test of side vision shows constriction, and it may be so bad as to give the impression of "tunnel vision," an incorrect term, but one which correctly implies severe restriction of peripheral vision.

Eventually the problem may become so bad so as to affect the cones of the macula also, leading to potential legal blindness, or rarely, almost complete blindness. It should be pointed out that a person may be considered legally blind due to visual field limitation alone, even if they could read the 20/40 line on the Snellen chart. There is no treatment, surgically or medically. Genetic counseling may detect if a person is likely to pass on the trait, and family members may need to be tested, even if apparently unaffected. Special low-vision aids may be helpful, and rehabilitation services are available for those severely affected, usually not until midlife. If hearing is also affected, the condition is called Usher's syndrome.

Keratoconus

The corneal window tissue of the eye is ideally spherical in curvature, like a smooth-surfaced round basketball. Astigmatism is an irregular curvature of the cornea, such that there is a long axis and a short axis of the cornea, like a spoon or the side of a football. Keratoconus means that the cornea (kerato) becomes cone shaped (conus), more like the pointed end of a football.

The signs of keratoconus usually begin in the late teens to the early twenties, more commonly in males, and are represented in the onset as an increase in nearsightedness or change of astigmatism, such that glasses need changing, often more frequently than convenient for annual checkups. When vision can no longer be satisfactorily corrected with spectacles, hard contact lenses may give quite good vision. Fitting of such contact lenses is difficult but is actually considered a treatment of the disease, such that it is about the only medical justification for fitting contact lenses, and in this case they must be hard contact lenses. For this reason, with the doctor's confirmation of this indication, medical insurance may cover the cost. The surface irregularity can be measured by a topography instrument, and this can be used to follow progress.

The reason hard contact lenses work is that a hard contact lens has its own spherical curvature, and thus the front contact lens surface bends or focuses light images undistorted onto the retina. Since the surface of the cornea is out of round, the tear layer is just of different thickness against the back surface of the contact lens. Hard contact lenses have thus always done a better job of correcting astigmatism, since a soft contact lens just lays on the cornea and takes up the same out-of-round curvature of the cornea. Therefore, the astigmatism is still present when a soft contact lens is worn. For comfort reasons, however, in the treatment of keratoconus, sometimes a piggyback fitting is created, whereby a hard contact lens is fit over the top of a soft contact lens.

Many people with keratoconus are already wearing contact lenses when the diagnosis is made, especially if nearsighted. The development of keratoconus in a hard contact lens wearer is sometimes suspected as being due to warpage of the cornea *caused* by the contact lens, so it is sometimes hard to tell which came first. Since the condition is supposed to be more common in males, the suspicion of contact lens cause of keratoconus is greater in a female contact lens wearer who develops signs of irregular astigmatism such as noted with keratoconus.

Because the natural course of keratoconus is to stop getting worse eventually, say between ages twenty-five and forty, the successful treatment with contact lenses usually persists. However, in some cases, inadequate correction of vision, complications in fitting contact lenses comfortably, or decompensation of the cornea may lead to the need for corneal transplantation.

Removing the cone-shaped central cornea and replacing it with a healthy donor cornea is usually quite successful. There still may be significant astigmatism postoperatively such that hard contact lenses again may be needed. The most important result, of course, is to restore good vision, and as has been mentioned, most keratoconus patients do not reach the stage of surgery.

EYE INJURIES

Blow to the Eye

Hyphema

This concussion injury is the most common traumatic eye injury needing attention. The injury may result from a finger to the eye, in sports, a tennis ball, or even a champagne cork. Blood, apparently due to a broken blood vessel in the iris tissue, flows in front of the pupil and covers part of the colored iris part of the eye. Due to gravity, naturally the blood shifts to the lower part of the eye. If, however, the level of blood is great enough, the pupil is covered, and a complete hyphema is possible, meaning neither the pupil nor the iris is visible.

A complete hyphema would be of more concern, since filling of the anterior chamber with blood means that the intraocular pressure would probably be increased. Blood, like aqueous fluid, can drain via the anterior chamber angle, but plugging of the system with thicker blood may result in increased intraocular pressure, even high enough to cause pain. Depending on how high the pressure has risen determines whether the treatment involves pressure-lowering medication or surgical drainage of the blood from the anterior chamber.

Treatment for hyphema was traditionally bed rest, with binocular occlusion for five days. Recurrent bleeding usually occurs within five days, during the stage of the so-called capillary fragility during which the blood vessels heal themselves. Cost of hospitalization versus little difference in results, has resulted in currently mainly outpatient treatment.

Other than bedrest, which can be varied per patient, topical eye drops to reduce the inflammation caused by the blood in the eye, and a medication called Amicar can be used to reduce the likelihood of recurrent hemorrhage. Daily office exams may be recommended. Rarely, surgical drainage of the blood from the anterior chamber of the eye may be needed, if the blood is not going away and potential complications, such as blood staining of the cornea, exist.

Black Eye

Any injury around the eye, such as a fist injury, causes bleeding under the skin and bruising called ecchymosis. The tissues around the eye are soft and swell easily. Therefore, a black eye, blood beneath the skin around the eye, may seem to spread. Often, to one's surprise, a black eye on one side of the nose can result in a black eye on the other side of the nose, because the skin on the nose is so tight and allows spread to the looser skin on the other side, causing a raccoon effect. Also, because of gravity, the last place for the blood to disappear is in the baggy part at the bottom of the lower eyelid. As blood slowly absorbs, a yellowish discoloration occurs. The main concern, naturally, is that a black eye may signify more serious injury to the eye itself, or the bones around the eye, suggesting need for an eye examination.

Ruptured Globe

This is the most serious injury and results from such things as a BB gun, rock, fingers, hand ball, or golf ball. Recognition of severity can be noted by swelling of the tissues around the eye, decreased vision, distortion of the pupil, and pain. A severe hyphema may signify serious injury, including laceration or rupture of the "globe," meaning a wound through the full thickness of the scleral cover or cornea, allowing intraocular fluids to leak out, and potential infection.

Emergency repair by an ophthalmologist is required, usually available to the call of an emergency room physician. Injuries may be so severe that authorization for removal of the injured eye should be obtained prior to surgery, rather than requiring a second surgery. Believe me, this is the last thing the ophthalmologist will want to do if he or she can avoid it.

Blow-Out Fracture

This orbital fracture results from a larger force such as a fist. A black eye, double vision, limitation of upward eye movement, and numbness of the skin of the upper lip suggest such a fracture. The eyeball itself may be uninjured. Repair, if it is an isolated injury, may be performed by an ophthalmologist. If accompanied by fractures of other bones of the face, it can be repaired by an ear, nose, and throat doctor, a plastic surgeon, or an oral surgeon.

Retinal Injury

a. Retinal detachment can occur from concussion injury, as seen with boxers. However, most retinal detachments are spontaneous. Surgical repair is usually urgent.

b. Commotio retinae is a term for the concussion injury of the retina, signified by retinal hemorrhages and transient or permanent loss of vision. Like any loss of vision following injury, this diagnosis requires examination by an eye doctor.

Eyelid Lacerations

This type injury can result from blunt or sharp instrument trauma. Wounds around the eye, eyelids, and brow can frequently be repaired by an emergency room physician. Lacerations involving the eyelid margin require repair by an ophthalmologist.

It is important to recognize the potential severity of lacerations, including dog bites, involving the part of the eyelid toward the nose. This is because such an injury may cut across the tear duct tissues and require special repair. This is to preserve the tear function, so that tears may drain normally from the eye. A pediatric or plastic surgical ophthalmologist may be required, and this is something that can usually wait until the next morning, or up to 48 hours to obtain such special services.

Foreign Bodies

A foreign object may be quite small but, if lodged under the upper eyelid, may be quite irritating. Usually the tearing of the eye will wash out most small foreign bodies unless embedded or held tightly against the eye by the upper eyelid. Then it may be necessary to flip or turn the upper lid so as to expose the undersurface to bring the foreign body into view. Sometimes it is so transparent that it is difficult to see, even with a slit lamp. When observing without magnification, it may be a good idea to swab across the undersurface of the eyelid with the hope of dislodging a foreign body not visible. Irrigation may also help by having the patient look down while irrigating under the upper eyelid. Relief is usually prompt, signifying success, but there may be residual irritation temporarily from scratches caused by rubbing on the cornea.

A corneal foreign body is common, especially involving a piece of iron, as associated by pounding or grinding on metal (fork-lift operators are also good candidates). The piece of metal, especially if hot, can stick to the cornea, and, if iron, can cause a rust ring reaction to the corneal tissue. Symptomatically, those with a corneal foreign body identify the problem as something under the upper eyelid, since blinking causes this reference. The doctor, from experience, knows that the first place to look is on the cornea, with a slit lamp.

Corneal foreign bodies, especially if a piece of hot iron embedded in the surface of the cornea, require removal with a relatively sharp instrument called a spud. If present for more than a few hours, a rust ring results from ferrous (iron) foreign bodies, and this must also be removed as well as possible. Sometimes the emergency room doctor can remove the foreign body, but, recognizing the presence of a rust ring, refers the patient to an ophthalmologist for definitive treatment. If not removed adequately, a rust ring may cause swelling to the point that the foreign body may seem to have come back. Such treatment need not be so scary, since topical eye drop medication can numb the eye so that only some reasonable cooperation allows treatment at with the slit lamp.

Following removal of the corneal object, there needs to be treatment of the resultant corneal abrasion. The surface of the cornea has to heal and will do so in a matter of hours. Eye drops may be prescribed to speed recovery without infection. A tiny scar may result, seldom affecting the vision if properly treated.

An intraocular foreign body can occur, and this is also usually metal. Sometimes a small piece of metal resulting from an explosion or similar force can penetrate the cornea or scleral coat of the eye and lodge inside the eye, in the retina. Seeing it through a dilated pupil can be helpful. Also, special X-ray techniques can help localize the object. Surgically, once localized, the object can be approached posteriorly by an incision made in the sclera overlying the object. If magnetic, a magnet can be applied over the incision and the magnetic foreign body can cut itself out through the soft tissues of the retina and choroid to attach itself to the magnetic tip. If other portions of the eye are not injured, vision may be restored. Untreated, however, most metallic foreign bodies would do damage to the eye in the process of degradation.

Chemical Injuries

Such injuries are quite common, and severity varies from minor to disastrous. The worst are due to alkaline injury, especially with something like powdered lye or lime. The main treatment is prompt irrigation, and in many cases this is all that is necessary. A shower, garden hose, or some of the now common bottles of water (squeezed so as to cause a stream) can be very helpful. More definitive treatment in the form of eye drops will be prescribed by the eye doctor. Sever alkaline burns may require hospitalization, and sometimes even a corneal transplant.

Strangely enough, glue is not so uncommonly a source of injury. The crazy-glue-like adhesive used for fingernails comes in a small bottle similar to that of eye drops. I can recall at least two patients who unwittingly reached into their purse and put what they thought were eye drops into their eye. The glue usually didn't injure the eye itself so much, due to blinking, but sure did glue the eyelashes together. The stronger upper-lid lashes overpower the lower lashes and pull them out, so that the eye can at least open. However, the lower lashes stick down, like fence posts hanging from the upper eyelashes. Being female, and embarrassed, neither patient returned for follow-up, and apparently took care of the problem herself. Eye ointments can help loosen glue.

First Aid and Prevention

As mentioned, irrigation of the eye, with caution, is indicated when it appears that dust or liquid chemical has splashed into the eye. Careful examination with a flashlight can help determine the severity of the injury. The natural tearing of the eye will wash out small particles, unless embedded in the cornea or trapped under the upper lid. Sometimes, by gentle traction downward, by pulling down the lashes of the upper lid over the lower lid, the lashes of the lower eyelid may help dislodge a particle stuck to the inner surface of the upper eyelid. The injured person will be able to tell relief promptly.

If there appears to be a laceration that may involve the eyeball, then the eye should be carefully covered and the patient transported to a hospital emergency room.

Prevention of injury usually involves the use of safety glasses, goggles, or shield. Safety glasses required by some types of work are heavier so as to provide more protection and can be prescription (sometimes paid for by the employer). Such glasses are usually so heavy that a person has another pair for regular use. Ordinary glasses, of course, provide some protection, certainly compared to those who wear no glasses. Contact lenses are also somewhat protective, for example, against foreign bodies, which might otherwise stick to the cornea.

Solar Injury to the Eyes

Ultraviolet (Short Wavelength) or UV Injury

UV injury to the eyes is common, for example, in arc welding, in suntan parlors, or as a complication of skiing (actinic keratitis). A welder usually knows better than to weld without a protective shield, but sometimes observers think they are safe if not too close and not looking at the work. Tanning booths insist on protective eyewear. A skier may be totally surprised that the injury is due to sunlight reflected off the snow, when inadequate sunglasses are worn. The surprise comes later, since there is no immediate discomfort so as to warn that an injury has occurred.

After an interval of hours, usually 6–12, and therefore frequently during the middle of the night, the injured person awakens with severe pain in the eyes. The eyelids are swollen and tightly closed. The eyes water, have scratchy foreign-body sensation, and photosensitivity. When examined by a doctor, the relief can be immediate if the doctor uses anesthetic eye drops in order to allow opening of the eyes for examination. The anesthetic drops numb the cornea, the swelling of which is the source of the pain. Unfortunately, the relief lasts only 30 minutes or so, then the medication wears off. A patient naturally wants some more of that good stuff, but unfortunately, repeated use of the anesthetic delays healing. A strong sedative sleeping pill will help get through the night, and relief will be rapid subsequently, such that complete recovery can be expected in 48 hours.

During the episode, patients feel blind but mainly because they cannot open their eyes, hence the term "snow blindness." Fortunately, there are no lasting aftereffects, which may be hard for someone to believe after so much discomfort. It is not unusual for a person to blame a subsequent eye problem on this episode. The pain is due to temporary swelling of the cornea, therefore a keratitis, and helps confirm that the cornea is the most pain-sensitive tissue in the body.

The normal lens of the eye absorbs UV so well that the retina is protected. Attempts have been made to duplicate this filtration ability by adding UV protection to the intraocular lens implants, with only limited success. Following cataract surgery, it is the extra ultraviolet reaching the retina that is responsible for the shift of color recognition as making everything look bluer, a shade that is usually not offensive, especially compared to the dimming of color recognition caused by the cataract that was removed. Exposure to too much sun has been felt to be a possible cause of cataracts, and such exposure to UV has experimentally produced cataracts in lab animals.

There are rare individuals who seem to develop corneal swelling after what would ordinarily be considered relatively minor sun exposure, such that relatively limited attacks are reported. These people need be extra careful in wearing sunglass protection. Also, anyone who has had cataract surgery needs to wear protective sunglasses, and usually is aware of more light sensitivity following surgery. Transition spectacle lenses, which darken automatically, can be a good choice in eyewear. Gray sunglasses seem to be preferable as a choice of tint due to the preservation of normal color appreciation. Polaroid sunglasses are the best in protection and are now available in prescription. Wraparound sunglasses are popular but are not available in prescription lenses.

Solar Retinopathy

This is most commonly a result of an eclipse burn from looking directly at the sun. Infrared (long wavelength) or IR light injury to the eye is rare, and it is debatable as to whether it is infrared IR or ultraviolet (short wavelength) UV radiation that causes solar retinopathy, or both. Ordinarily, the retina is protected from solar injury because a person reflexively looks away from the sun when it is too bright. There are reports of druggies so spaced out that they looked at the sun too long, or of religious fanatics doing so on purpose. The danger with an eclipse is that the moon covers enough of the sun such that one can look more directly at the solar source, perhaps long enough to create a burn in the retina. Since the macula is the focal point of vision, this damage results in loss of reading vision. There are reports of solar retinopathy with lesser exposure, and there are also reports of spontaneous recovery. However, it is too much of a risk to look at an eclipse, even with protective shielding.

There is also the story of the soldier involved in nuclear experimentation in the early stages. Supposedly, his unit was to hide in a trench at a distance thought perhaps safe from radiation injury. Though told to cover his eyes, this man reportedly stood up, opened one eye, and saw the mushroom cloud of the blast. His retina showed an upside-down mushroom scar of the macula, because, of course, things are reversed upside down in the eye, and explaining why he lost vision in that eye.

17

THINGS TO KNOW ABOUT EYE SURGERY

Eye surgery has been discussed in a discussion of diseases requiring surgery, but perhaps some details of eye surgery would be interesting. For example, just what happens, and what can you expect if you are the patient. And no, we do not take the eye out, operate on it, and put it back in place.

CATARACT SURGERY

Cataract surgery, as mentioned, is the most common surgical procedure performed in the United States, and perhaps all countries. The surgical procedure has enjoyed many improvements in recent years. Removal of the lens of the eye was performed by rather relatively gross techniques years ago, and the introduction of sutures meant better and more rapid postoperative improvement. By the 1940s to 1950s, the lens of the eye was removed in one piece (intracapsular cataract extraction). Then a technique called Kelman phacoemulsification arose in the 1970s, utilizing a very small incision. This is a form of "extracapsular" cataract extraction, meaning that all the lens is removed, except for the capsular envelope that surrounds the soft internal portion of the lens, a tissue like cellophane. This allows an envelope sort of arrangement into which the intraocular lens (IOL) implant could fit into proper position. Contrary to common belief, this phacoemulsification does not involve laser, but instead involves ultrasound.

There are different techniques, and you may wish to discuss with your surgeon just what he does. By the way, I use the male gender when discussing eye doctors, realizing that almost half of the eye doctors being trained are female. Cataract surgery is an outpatient procedure. There is no such thing as being too old to have the surgery, and almost no such thing as being too sick. It takes about 2 hours in the outpatient surgicenter. It also is not a reason to postpone surgery, because of fear of the unknown. This fear can usually be lessened by good information. The procedure almost always is done under local anesthesia, meaning an anesthesiologist is there to help, but it is not necessary to be put to sleep. You probably will not even remember what happens, even though if asked a question during the surgery, you may be able to respond. Once, when I was standing next to my patient postoperatively in the recovery room, her daughter came in, and the patient said, "They didn't do my surgery." So if you insist on worrying about your surgery, you can be sure that all the worry will be gone once the anesthesia doctor starts working.

The eye is numbed, but now days this can be done topically, meaning with eye drops and an injection of numbing medicine once the eye is open. A small incision is made in the cornea, one so small that usually no sutures are needed. Small tubular instruments are inserted, and a round incision is made in the front surface of the lens, a capsulotomy. Then all the lens cortex and nucleus is removed, by ultrasound, irrigation, and aspiration (suction). A flexible foldable intraocular lens is implanted (inserted) into the capsular space, like into an envelope, with the opening being (the capsulotomy) in the front of what was the lens of the eye.

When awakened, the relaxing medicine having worn off, the patient can soon go home. At home, one is not confined to bed but can sit and watch TV. There may be an eye pad over the eye and/or a protective shield, but if only a shield, one can see right away through the holes of the shield. Eye drops of anti-inflammatory nature are taken, and usually the next day in the doctor's office, patients can get an early idea of how well they are going to see. Things look brighter and whiter, actually due to the Purkinje shift, meaning that more of the blue end of the light spectrum is getting into the eye. This is because the natural lens of the eye is better at filtering out ultraviolet light than any intraocular lens implant, but it's OK, everything looks brighter.

Restrictions of activity are minimal, and the doctor may allow return to work soon, depending on the nature of work. Since most patients are seniors, regular activities are usually allowed, and any needed glasses can be prescribed in about three weeks. If temporary reading glasses are needed, the doctor can suggest what to get at the drug store. If an accommodative or pseudoaccommodative implant is used, the procedure and follow-up is pretty much the same.

I actually heard an ad over the radio once for some vitamins that were to prevent cataracts, of course, which is ridiculous. The funniest part was a statement that if you have cataract surgery, it just might grow back. This statement, though incorrect, requires comment, because there is such a thing as a "secondary cataract." The back surface of the capsule, the membrane left intact, which was the original cellophane-like wrapper of the original lens of the eye, may become clouded at some point after surgery. As it becomes clouded, it represents a blur to the eye because less light is getting through the pupil, like when the original cataract was developing. This may give the impression that the cataract is coming back. If enough of a nuisance, the treatment is simple and painless. This is where a laser is actually used in cataract treatment. A "Yag" laser, attached to a slit lamp microscope, can be focused onto this membrane and a hole popped through the clouded capsule, kind of like a pupil behind the pupil, and light comes through the IOL again clearly. Instant return to good vision results.

The question comes up as to where one should go to have cataract surgery and whether to go to a surgeon who one has heard does a whole lot of cataracts, and is a cataract specialist. Certainly in our field, some high-volume cataract surgeons have evolved. I would suggest that if you have a local ophthalmologist with whom you have developed a good relationship, and you know of patients who have received good results and care from this doctor, that it would probably be better to stay with your doctor for the surgery. A different doctor, depending on location and other factors, may be glad to oblige doing the surgery, but not wish or be able to give you the kind of continued follow-up care you should have. Often, after going out of town for the surgery, patients are embarrassed to return to the care of their original doctor. As result, they may not get examinations as frequently as suggested and may even resort to inadequate glasses such as drug store glasses, or go to some other stranger for care. A general rule is that anyone having undergone cataract surgery should be examined at least once a year. There may not be any complications of the cataract surgery, but other problems also need possible detection. Of course, the second eye is a question regarding health and cataract.

GLAUCOMA SURGERY

In discussing the treatment of glaucoma, surgery was mentioned as the treatment one seeks when treatment of pressure-lowering eye drops or laser treatment has not provided adequate control of the intraocular pressure.

The simplest surgery is the iridectomy performed for angle closure glaucoma. This was once done surgically as an outpatient procedure. In recent years, this has been done with a laser, and really not an invasive surgical procedure, being rather quick and safe. The indication would be an attack of angle closure glaucoma, or recognition of the same potential for an attack in the other eye. The real issue is prophylactic or preventive treatment of a patient whose anterior chamber angles seem narrow via microscopic gon-ioscopy.

The anterior chamber depth is estimated first by slit lamp microscopic examination, and is expectedly more narrow in the farsighted eye, which is anatomically smaller. A special examination by a gonioscope lens can show whether there is much space between the root of the iris and the ciliary body, rather like looking around the corner. If the space seems quite narrow, then there is concern that an attack of angle closure glaucoma may occur. This stimulates the idea of preventive therapy, either with pilocarpine drops, which shrink the pupil so as to widen the anterior chamber angle, or with laser iridotomy to make an extra pupil for easy access of fluid to the anterior chamber angle drainage area. People are attracted to a quick fix, such that the laser alternative seems best. Nevertheless, eye doctors frequently place their patients on pilocarpine even after laser iridotomy. In spite of all this concern,

I am not personally aware of anyone who suffered an attack of angle closure glaucoma after either means of preventive treatment.

An intermediate treatment of open-angle glaucoma, when eye drop therapy has failed, or because, again, people are interested in a quick fix, is laser trabeculoplasty. Some debate whether this is really surgery, but it is relatively simple and without much complication. The biggest complication is that it may not work to continued satisfaction or for very long. What is involved is a laser burn placed in the chamber angle tissue called the trabecular meshwork, which is the filtering area through which fluid drains from the eye into veins. It is rather a plumbing approach to improve the outflow. If this does not work, it can be repeated. However, it is not unusual to have to resort to the use of glaucoma eye drops to supplement future treatment. Newer lasers have better potential results and allow less limited repeated procedures if necessary.

Glaucoma surgery amounts to methods to drain fluid from the eye, in a controlled fashion, so as to lower the intraocular pressure to safe ranges. There are different methods based on making an improvement of fluid release from the eye. Trabeculectomy amounts to making a surgical wedge opening into the anterior chamber angle, and purposely creating reasons why this opening should remain open, such as taking out some tissue. In in other words, creating a wound that does not heal completely. Filtration is encouraged through the sclera and under the conjunctiva, creating what is called a bleb, which is like a blister containing aqueous fluid, which can eventually be drained in a controlled fashion by veins from the eye.

Complications include possible infection, failure to filter enough fluid, or even filtering too much fluid. Failures can sometimes be salvaged by needling the bleb, or reoperations. The use of glaucoma drops may also be needed eventually to maximize effect. Apparent early success may be complicated by eventual scarring down of the bleb.

Other surgical approaches involve a stint, tube, or shunt with artificial implanted material, which encourages filtration of fluid, like a wick under the conjunctiva, to form a bleb, or a direct drainage into a space inside the choroid. These procedures may be necessary if the conjunctiva is scarred from previous surgery such as a cataract operation.

From the patient standpoint, the experience would be similar to outpatient cataract surgery. An anesthesiologist makes the experience forgetful, and postoperative discomfort is expected to be minimal. Of course follow-up is very important to see if the treatment is successful or if further treatment is needed.

As far as where to go for surgery, this is something your general ophthalmologist will help decide with you. Glaucoma specialists have evolved, having had special training in treating glaucoma. Most general ophthalmologists do not do the filtering-type surgical procedures for glaucoma, though some may do laser treatments. As a rule, when it is determined that eye drop topical therapy is not successful, then by mutual decision, referral to a glaucoma specialist is recommended, if available. The patient is then referred back to the general primary ophthalmologist eventually for continued follow-up, and sometimes further use of topical eye drop therapy is needed. It seems to be true that glaucoma specialists are mainly interested in procedures and are not likely to want to conduct the indefinitely long follow-up required for glaucoma patients, including checking vision and detecting other problems in the course of routine comprehensive examinations. Some patients are interested in a "quick fix" and may be too impatient to take long-term topical therapy. They may seek out a glaucoma specialist who will perform a laser procedure, or filtering surgery, so as to avoid the need to use eye drops. However, early good results are sometimes only temporary, and if the patients are too embarrassed to return to their original primary ophthalmologist, they may actually lose vision from an undiagnosed return of high pressure, inadequate visual correction, or un-detected eye disease. Probably, if such patients would disclose their intent, to shortcut the use of annoying eye drops, their eye doctor would probably sup-port them in their decision, and agree to take over their care upon completion of treatment by the glaucoma specialist.

RETINAL DETACHMENT SURGERY

A retinal detachment can be serious and can require sometimes emergency treatment surgically. The incidence is reported as one for every 10,000 people per year. Though this seems a small incidence, the consequences can be devastating. Detachment of the retina is more common in higher degrees of myopia (nearsightedness) and also following cataract extraction. The retina lines the back of the eye and has been likened to the film in the back of a camera. It is delicate nerve tissue and is like wallpaper in how it lines the back of the eye. A hole in the retina can occur, sometimes from trauma, but usually spontaneously. Thinking of the eye like a room filled with fluids, if a hole forms in the retina, it is like a hole in wallpaper. The fluid can get into the hole and wash away the retina, like wallpaper stripping from the side of a room. Gravity plays a role such that a hole high up in the eye is more likely to allow fluid to enter and strip away the retina. However, a hole lower in the eye is slower in progress to strip away the retina, like would be unlikely with the antigravitational effect of a hole in wallpaper near the bottom of a room.

The macula, as has been described, is very special and delicate. If the macula is detached, or stripped away from its usual location, the prognosis is poor for recovery of good vision. It is like having thousands of little electrical plugs unplugged and trying to realign these tiny plugs with repair of the retinal detachment. Thus what may appear to be a good anatomical result may not be a good functional result, if the macula is detached in the process.

Surgical repair of a retinal detachment is major surgery in most cases. A general anesthetic is usually required, though the procedure can be done under local anesthesia. Also, it is more likely to be an inpatient procedure, requiring overnight stay in the hospital. For a significant detachment, what is called a scleral buckle is usually involved. This means that the hole in the retina is identified and localized. Then a band is placed around the eye so as to elevate the tissue beneath the hole. Then, when the fluid is drained from beneath the retina, it drapes onto the buckle as it falls back in place. Treatment to the tissue forming the buckle in the form of heat or laser creates a sticky reaction that helps seal the retina in place. If all goes well, then the retina stays in place, and depending on whether the macula was involved, vision may be fully restored. However, the buckle is like a belt around the eye, and it tends to make the eye longer than originally, and therefore more relatively nearsighted.

Once satisfactorily treated, the retinal hole causing the problem is firmly sealed and not likely to cause further trouble. Nearsighted people are more likely to develop a retinal detachment. This is because the nearsighted or myopic eye is larger than average, and, if highly nearsighted, has retinal tissue rather stretched out to line the back of the eye. Holes in the retina therefore occur more spontaneously in highly nearsighted eyes. Cataract surgery increases the likelihood of retinal detachment, and therefore the idea of performing "presbyopia surgery" on a highly nearsighted person who doesn't even have a cataract raises alertness to possible retinal detachment complication.

There are other methods of treating a retinal detachment. Sometimes injection of a gas into the vitreous can force the retina back in place, a pneumatic retinopexy. Treatment like such as spot welding, with laser, can then help hold the retina in place. Sometimes this sort of treatment can be performed in the office. If the vitreous is filled with blood, or if the vitreous seems to be a factor in pulling off the retina, a surgical vitrectomy may need to be performed with an operating microscope. Also vitrectomy can be employed in stripping off a membrane causing preretinal macular fibrosis. Laser treatment can also be applied to needed areas to help stick the retina in place endoscopically (from the inside via the use of the operating microscope).

The other eye of course needs to be closely watched, since it also has increased likelihood of retinal detachment. Also, other members of the family, especially if also nearsighted, need to be watched carefully for signs of retinal detachment. Areas of retinal thinning or degeneration, such as "lattice degeneration," may be treated prophylactically with laser. Symptoms, as mentioned in the discussion of floaters and flashes, should be attended to by careful retinal examination. Even if the exam is normal, further symptoms of a shower of floaters, or a shadow in any field of vision, should indicate a need for further exam.

Retinal detachments are usually detected by primary ophthalmologists or optometrists, with a referral to a retinal specialist ophthalmologist. It is not necessary to see a retinal specialist for routine exams if you are a diabetic, or for symptoms of floaters or flashes. A screening exam can be performed by your primary eye doctor, and then a referral will be recommended depending on the need. After retinal surgery or treatment, a period of follow-up will be suggested by the retinal doctor, but the patient will be referred back to the primary eye doctor for long-term follow-up.

STRABISMUS SURGERY

Surgery on eye muscles is usually performed on children who are cross-eyed. The surgery is not as difficult as intraocular surgery such as cataract surgery. Preoperative recognition of what needs to done and designing the surgery for each patient is what is more difficult. One of my professors, Dr. Fred Blodi, used to say, "I can teach a monkey to operate. The question is when." Other methods of treating crossed eyes need to be employed first, glasses if indicated (usually), and elimination of amblyopia (lazy eye) if possible.

I believe, and some agree with me, that the incidence of surgery for cross-eyed children is less than it was, because there are fewer cross-eyed children. Why, I don't know. Most general ophthalmologists once performed such "muscle" surgery. Currently, this type of surgery is almost always done by pediatric ophthalmologists who have specialized training. This is true for adults who need strabismus surgery also, since general ophthalmologists have stopped doing such operations. I know a professional football player named Mike, who was greeted in the waiting room of a pediatric ophthalmologist, a friend of mine, to whom he was referred. The nurse came into the waiting room, looking around for a boy and saying, "Mikey, Mikey, it's your turn Mikey," only to be startled by a 6-foot-3-inch man weighing 285 pounds, arising and saying, "I am Mikey."

As described, eye muscle surgery utilizes somewhat orthopedic principles (carpentry) to a neurological (electronic) problem. The rectus muscles, which rotate the eyes, are estimated to be 100 times more powerful than necessary for the work they do. They work in coordinated synchrony. When the muscle that turns the eye toward the nose is active, the medial rectus, the opposing muscle, which is to rotate the eye toward the ear, the lateral rectus, must relax and stretch. It is rarely true that a cross-eyed child has any weak eye muscles.

The eye that crosses all the time, is frequently called the "weak eye," but this is not true, it is not weak. The other eye has just become the preferred eye, and this may have resulted from the fact that the crossed eye does not see as well and is amblyopic. When surgery is done, it could be on either eye, and this is difficult for parents to understand, largely because they like to think that the surgery will make the "weak eye" stronger. With this in mind, the eye surgeon routinely operates on the eye that is usually crossed. However, if reoperation due to incomplete success in the first operation is indicated, it is certainly more logical to work on the other eye, even if it is the better-seeing or preferred eye. Scar tissue from the first operation makes it more difficult to estimate the results of the second operation if done on the same eye as the first operation. Another factor, is that there is a limit to what can be done to a given muscle, and if the maximum has been done already, then obviously the other eye must be used in the second surgery.

For the cross-eyed patient, the medial rectus, the muscle that turns the eye in toward the nose, is recessed (set back) or weakened in its effect. Sometimes both medial rectus muscles are recessed, and seldom is only one muscle operated upon. Usually, along with recessing one medical rectus muscle, the lateral rectus in the same eye is resected, or tightened so as to have more effect. This can be painful under local anesthesia, which some adults request, and since most cross-eyed patients who have surgery are children, a general anesthetic is usually used. It still can be an outpatient procedure.

For exotropia, out-turning of one the eye, the decision for surgery may not come until beyond childhood. Most commonly both lateral rectus muscles are recessed (set back) or weakened in effect. Sometimes the medial rectus is resected or shortened in one eye. One of the frequent indications for exotropia surgery is a complication of prior surgery for esotropia, called consecutive exotropia. This is especially the case if the amount of surgery for crossing of the eyes is based on the amount of crossing present without glasses. A temporary good result is followed by later recognition of the need for glasses, and then out-turning of one eye, usually the eye operated upon. This type of reoperation is complicated by the scar tissue from the first operation. Strangely enough, the best lasting result from surgery for primary exotropia, whereby the patient has the ability to ignore the image of one eye when it drifts out but retains a form of binocular vision most of the time, is to see temporarily double after the surgery due to being a little cross-eyed. Since the natural tendency is to drift more outward with time, this transient double vision helps develop a more lasting binocular result.

Vertical muscle surgery is less common. Results are less predictable, and usually the amounts of surgery needed are relatively small. One indication is to release the tightness of the inferior rectus, the muscle that pulls the eye down, when affected by hyperthyroidism or blowout orbital fracture, so that the eye can look upward better.

CORNEAL TRANSPLANT

The cornea is the only part of the eye that can be transplanted. It is also unusual in that, contrary to other transplantable organs, it is not necessary to cross-match with the donor. The donor is usually someone who, before death, agreed to donate their eyes for the use of their corneas to help someone regain their sight. Donated eyes are transported in refrigerated storage, often by the highway patrol, and kept at an eye bank for distribution to requesting hospitals, usually in urgent response. If you can imagine, sometimes the highway patrol from one state hands the container across the state line to the highway patrol of the neighboring state, a true relay team.

The surgery is done under local anesthesia and takes an hour or so. A cookie-cutter type surgical trephine is used to remove the center of the patient's diseased cornea, and an identical portion of the donor cornea is removed. Then the donor "graft" is sutured into place by microfine sutures, which can be left in place for a long period of time. New exciting techniques are being developed to make the donor and recipient graft tissues match more exactly, so as to give better visual result.

Postoperatively the patient must protect the eye. Vision may be immediately improved, depending on the preoperative problem, but the visual results may not be fully recognized for many months. Topical steroid eye drops may be needed for a long time to avoid rejection or failure of the graft.

A contact lens may be needed to give the best vision after a corneal transplant. The sutures may need removal in stages. If the graft is rejected, it can be replaced by another transplant. The success rate is high, perhaps 90 percent, and new techniques of trephination and suturing are being utilized to give even better results.

A corneal specialist would perform the surgery and be involved in follow-up for a long time. However, general eye care will be referred back to the primary eye doctor.

ENUCLEATION

Sometimes the eye becomes so sick it needs to be removed, and this is called enucleation. Sometimes enucleation is because of a tumor such as a melanoma. The thought of this is, of course, quite depressing. But sometimes, the removal of the eye is preferable for comfort or cosmetic reasons. A badly injured or diseased eye tends to shrink and become abnormal in appearance. As a rule, if an eye has no sight, has no potential sight, and is painful, then it should be removed, especially if unsightly. The elimination of the pain and the discomfort of a deformed eye can be very helpful to a patient. When an eye loses its sight, in adult life, it turns outward. Should this happen in childhood, it would cross and then later in adult life drift outward. In addition to not being straight, a badly damaged eye tends to shrink, called phthisis. Then the eyelids on that side droop. The eye may appear gray if the cornea is clouded or red if it is inflamed and painful.

Once a decision is made to remove an eye, there is reason for expectations of a positive result. An artificial eye is less objectionable and can be made to look fairly normal. The simplest procedure is to remove the eye and put a plastic ball in the space left empty. Another method, called evisceration, involves removing most, but not all, of the eye, and this can give good motility of a prosthesis later, since the muscles are left intact. Removal of the eye can be performed with orbital implant, meaning that a prosthetic implant is placed in the orbital space left empty by eye removal, usually with rotation causing muscles intact, and giving better cosmetic result.

There are prosthetics that include fixation of the extraocular muscles so as to give more normal-appearing movement of the prosthesis. Actually, the orbital implant is buried beneath the conjunctival layer, giving a pink look to the tissue. The prosthesis is then fit into place, like a big contact lens, over the implant. Movement of the orbital implant transmits friction to the overlying prosthesis and, depending on the type of implant, may give relatively normal movement of the prosthesis. The fitting of a prosthesis is by an "ocularist," and this can be quite an art. The cosmetic results can be quite good, so that it may be difficult to notice imperfect eye appearance or variance from movement of the other eye. Even if imperfect, the appearance of an artificial eye can be an improvement over a blind, unsightly eye.

A rare, but not insignificant, reason to remove an eye is that if a penetrating wound into the eye involves uveal tissue (the iris, ciliary body, or choroid), then there may develop an unusual form of uveitis, called sympathetic ophthalmia. For reasons yet unknown, the inflammation in the injured eye may spread to involve the uninjured eye, with disastrous potential effects, and is an indication to remove the eye at the time of injury if recognized that damage to the eye is so severe as to raise this prospect.

PART V

CONSUMER INFORMATION

18

DEFINITIONS OF CAREGIVERS

If you need advice, you can often depend on recommendations of friends or your primary physician. Whether you should go to an optometrist or an ophthalmologist might depend on your understanding of the difference. So what is the difference? And who is the person who makes glasses? The following are some definitions:

CAREGIVERS

Ophthalmologist

An ophthalmologist is a doctor of medicine (MD), a physician who completed a premed degree of usually four years, four years of medical school, an internship year, and three or four years of specialized training in ophthalmology, called a residency. This totals twelve or thirteen years of training, and also requires state licensure to practice medicine. Ophthalmologists specialize in treating all forms of eye disease, medical or surgical, anything from prescribing glasses, treating "pink eye," or performing surgery such as repairing injured eyes, or cataracts. Upon completion of satisfactory training, ophthalmologists are certified by the Board of Ophthalmology, having completed successfully written and oral testing. Recertification is now required, helping to assure that practicing ophthalmologists are current in information. Many hospitals require board certification in order to receive surgical privileges.

Those, like myself, are called general ophthalmologists. When I first practiced, that meant that we did everything, including all kinds of surgery, from retinal detachment, to strabismus and, plastic procedures such as blepharoplasty, glaucoma surgery, and so on. More recently, subspecialties, requiring an additional one to three years of additional training have evolved. These include pediatric, retinal, corneal and external disease, neuro-ophthalmic, glaucoma, oculoplastic, and now refractive surgery subspecialties. General ophthalmologists continue to treat all eye conditions, but surgically mainly operate on cataracts. Leadership is via the American Academy of Ophthalmology, which has suggested that ophthalmologists refer to themselves as Eye MDs, so as to avoid confusion with optometrists. Confusion about the difference has been a problem in the past.

Optometrist

An optometrist is an eye doctor who has completed three or four years of preoptometry training, much like predental training, and then four years of optometry school learning about eye disease. Optometrists also receive training in basic sciences, like medical students do, but to a lesser degree, again more like dentists get in their schooling. They have state licensure examinations and must be approved by the State Board of Optometry for relicensure, about every three years. Their training follows general medical principles, and as result, they are in agreement with the basics shared by ophthalmologists. Treatment historically was limited to evaluating vision, prescribing glasses and contact lenses, and detecting diseases requiring treatment by an ophthalmologist. More recently, partly because of the ambitious aims of organized optometry (American Optometry Association), practical needs, insurance, and the managed care industry, optometrists have sought, and received approval for, the treatment of many eye diseases such as conjunctivitis (pink eye), foreign bodies, and even glaucoma. Most recently, organized optometry has threatened to demand permission to perform eye surgery also. Certain states, such as Oklahoma and New Mexico, have considered approving this, though the actual practice of surgery by optometrists seems illogical. Laser surgery is an area of interest because it is essentially not hands-on cutting surgery, something for which they would be poorly trained (cataract surgery, for example). The scope of practice (privileges) for optometrists is determined by state legislatures, not a board of medicine. This is similar to chiropractors and podiatrists, whose scope of practice is also determined by state legislatures. For this reason, some states grant more privileges than others, and the scope of practice varies among optometrists of different states, meaning that the authorization to treat glaucoma or other diseases is not standardized. In general, optometry training is progressively better and comprehensive. Some schools train their students to be able to conform to the optometry scope of practice levels of any state in the country.

Optician

This person is licensed to dispense and fit glasses, utilizing a prescription from an optometrist or an ophthalmologist. Training results from a one to two year opticionary degree, or a two-year apprenticeship. State licensure is required in twenty-one states, and recertification via the American Board of Opticianry is every three years. For performing contact lens fitting, a special license is required. Opticians work in an optical shop, which may be freestanding, but more commonly owned by employing optometrists, ophthalmologists, or chain optical shops, such as Pearle Vision or Lens Crafters. Freestanding optical shops are now rare, since it became necessary for most ophthalmologists to dispense glasses in their offices. Chain optical shops and retail stores also employ optometrists, such as Wal-Mart, Sears, or Costco. Contact lenses are often fit in chain optical shops, and prices for the replacement of soft contact lenses are often low enough to attract patient prescriptions obtainable from their eye doctor.

Opticians take a spectacle prescription, measure the needed centration of lenses, depending on the frame selected, order the lenses from an optical lab, help select and fit frames, and often make simple repairs to glasses. It may be helpful for a patient to know that there is a difference in prescriptions. Ophthalmologists tend to write their prescriptions in what is called plus cylinders, whereas optometrists tend to write theirs in minus cylinders. The difference has to do with refracting technique and instruments. An optician converts all plus cylinder prescriptions to minus cylinder because that is the way the optical lab wants it. The patient, however, seeing a prescription from one doctor, say, an optometrist, and then comparing it to a newer prescription from an ophthalmologist may think someone has made a big mistake. For example, a prescription of -1.00 -1.00 axis 90 degrees converts to $-2.00 + 1.00$ axis 180 degrees; in other words they are identical prescriptions. So don't panic; just ask your doctor or the optician if concerned about a big apparent difference in prescriptions.

Another source of confusion regarding the eye doctor's glasses prescription is the so called "add," which refers to the reading addition. Someone looking at their prescription and seeing $+2.50$ add may think that the drug store appropriate glasses would be a $+2.50$. Actually, one must take into account the astigmatism, and also the sphere. For example, a person 1 diopter nearsighted would have -1.00 in the top part of the prescription, the "sphere." This must be combined with the $+2.50$ reading addition, and the result converts to a $+1.50$ reading glass at the drug store. The astigmatism factor, if significant, means there is no drug store equivalent.

Orthoptist

This technician is trained to deal with problems associated with strabismus and amblyopia, involving diagnosis and treatment. Because orthoptists work with eye exercises, sometimes there is confusion about their role in eye care. However, orthoptists are not those who claim to be able to help avoid the need for glasses by exercises, as advertised sometimes over the radio. They work usually with an ophthalmologist in strabismus management. Their chief therapeutic success with exercises is with the condition called convergence insufficiency, problems with bringing the eyes together for reading.

Ocularist

This specialist fits artificial eyes and can be quite skilled. Once the prosthesis is fitted, he or she needs to be consulted for follow-up cleaning and alterations routinely.

Ophthalmic Technician

These certified trained technicians assist an ophthalmologist in examinations and treatments in the doctor's office. In some states, they apparently can write a prescription for glasses, as a physician assistant. In other states, optometrists have legislated reduced privileges for such assistants.

Optometric Technician

These technicians are trained to assist an optometrist in examinations and treatments of eye disease and are usually certified following appropriate training.

With these defined roles, then it should be simple to answer questions of where to go for eye care, but it is not always so. All these professionals are designed to work together, and usually do, but there is a nonpublicized war going on between organized optometry and organized ophthalmology. It's a turf war, and about money and power, like most wars. Actually, this is no longer such a secret. See the January 31 issue of *U.S. News and World Report* discussing nonphysician clinicians. Also discussed in this issue are other nonphysician clinicians, such as physician assistants, nurse practitioners, oral surgeons, podiatrists, psychologists, and chiropractors. Along with optometrists, the changing role of these clinicians relative to the role of the physician is discussed. However, there is no question that the qualified role of the optometrist in helping ophthalmologists in eye care is unequaled by other "nonphysician clinicians."

Back in the times when their functions were limited to prescribing glasses and contact lenses, optometrists were quick to refer their patients to ophthalmologists for eye disease. Years ago ophthalmologists did not dispense glasses; it was considered unethical, so they prescribed glasses to be dispensed by optical shops. Later, it became desirable, and eventually required for ophthalmologists to dispense glasses. In the meantime, patients referred to an ophthalmologist often did not return to the referring optometrist, and stayed in the care of the ophthalmologist, for glasses too. Loss of patients, of course, made optometrists less interested in referring patients to ophthalmologists. Optometry schools began to emphasize treatment of ocular diseases, and legislators were successfully recruited to vote increased therapeutic privileges for optometrists in all states, one by one, but seldom the same privileges.

A current area of conflict between the two groups of eye doctors is the issue of "comanagement." In the case of cataract surgery, referring optometrists have insisted upon, or have been offered as inducement for referral, the approval of the operating surgeon for delegation of postoperative management of cataract patients by the referring doctor. In some cases, this was justified by allowing the patient to travel out of town for outpatient surgery and return home for postoperative care by their optometrist. In other cases, in a larger city, it was a condition of referral to a local ophthalmologist. The arrangement is not considered fee splitting, since postoperative care amounts to several visits, and comanagement is approved by insurance and Medicare. Some ophthalmologists refuse to agree to this arrangement, feeling optometrists are not suitably trained to recognize and treat complications, and that they, as surgeons, are ultimately responsible for surgical results. A more recent, and less disputed, area of comanagement is in refractive surgery. Refractive surgeons are very much motivated to encourage referrals, and actually are not set up to provide postoperative care for the volume of patients they seek. Follow-up by referring optometrist or ophthalmologist is usually satisfactory to the patient, with a referral back to the refractive surgeon for problems or revisions.

19

MORE THINGS YOU NEED TO KNOW

COMMON EYE DROP MEDICATIONS

We should review the manner in which one should instill eye drops into the eye. Of course it is easier if someone else puts the drops in, but even then there are some clues to making it easier. It is important to keep both eyes open when receiving eye drops, whether self-introduced or from a caregiver. Place the eye dropper over the eye to be treated, pull the lower eyelid downward, and look upward with both eyes. Then squeeze the bottle, aiming anywhere between the eyelids. If you feel the eye drop, then one drop is all that is required. However, if the drop runs down your face, or you think you missed, then put in another drop. If you want to prolong the action, or avoid side effects from the medicine running down the nose, where it may be absorbed into the blood stream, place the thumb and forefinger on each side of the nose between the eyes for a few seconds.

Examination Eye Drops

Anesthetic Eye Drops

Anesthetic eye drops, such as tetracaine or proparacaine, work instantly to numb the cornea for the purpose of measuring intraocular pressure or for relief of corneal pain, long enough to allow examination or treatment, such as removal of a corneal foreign body. Repeated use, however, can be toxic to the corneal surface epithelium, so these anesthetics cannot be dispensed to the patient.

Dyes

Dyes, such as flourescein, can be used topically to help identify scratches of the cornea, corneal erosions, punctate keratitis associated with viral infection, or the advanced stage of dry eye (keratoconjunctivitis sicca). Flourescein can also be injected intravenously for angiogram photographic examinations of the retina for the diagnosis of macular degeneration or diabetic retinopathy.

Mydriatics

Mydriatics are used to dilate the pupil, and short-acting ones are used to examine the retina in the course of routine comprehensive eye examinations. These wear off in a matter of minutes, during which time it is advisable to wear sunglasses outdoors. Focusing ability is temporarily weakened. Stronger long-acting dilating drops, the most common being atropine, are called cycloplegics because they temporarily paralyze or weaken the focusing muscles, while dilating the pupil. An atropine refraction exam is used in children who are cross-eyed or too young to be able to cooperate for examination. Atropine is also used as a form of patching of the good eye to force the use of the amblyopic (lazy) eye. Therapeutically, atropine is important in the treatment of significant iritis, to put the pupil at rest.

Anti-infectious Agents

Antibiotics

Antibiotics are used in drop form more than ointment form because ointments blur vision, can be messy, and sometimes delay healing. Sulfa, one of the original antibiotics, is still good, can be generic, and therefore less expensive. However, there is an increased incidence of sulfa allergies compared to newer antibiotics. Neomycin, usually in combination with bacitracin and polymyxin (Neosporin), is broad spectrum and effective, and also available over the counter (without prescription) in ointment form. However, neomycin used topically is most commonly likely to cause allergies such as contact dermatitis, estimated as 15–20 percent incidence.

Newer topical antibiotics are continuously becoming available, such as tobramycin (Tobrex) and flouroquinolones such as Cilox, Zymar, Quixin, Vigamox, and Ocuflox. Oral antibiotics are rarely necessary for the treatment of common infections such as conjunctivitis (pink eye). However, for some problems, such as stubborn blepharitis, tetracycline is employed. Tear duct infections or orbital infections may require oral antibiotics.

Treatment of most conjunctivitis involves the use of topical antibiotic drops, even though they do no good in the treatment of viral infection. It is difficult to detect whether an infection is viral or bacterial initially. Failure to respond and requirement of about a two-week course suggest a viral cause, whereas rapid resolution may indicate bacterial infection blunted by the antibiotic.

Antiviral Agents

Antiviral agents are used to treat herpetic infections. For herpes simplex (cold sore virus), topical Viroptic drops (or Stoxil), or ointments, such as Vira

A or Stoxil, will speed recovery. However, these topical medications are somewhat irritating, and their use needs to be titrated or cut back as soon as they are no longer needed. Oral acyclovir is helpful in treating either herpes simplex virus (HSV) or herpes zoster virus (HZV) infections and has minimal side effects.

Antifungal Medications

Antifungal medications fortunately are rarely necessary, but may be required topically for corneal ulcers or systemically for intraocular infections.

Anti-inflammatory Agents

Corticosteroids

Corticosteroids are used extensively in the treatment of eye inflammation, for allergy, iridocyclitis (inflammation of the iris or ciliary body), episcleritis (inflammation beneath the conjunctiva), scleritis (inflammation of the deeper white of the eye), and many kinds of keratitis (corneal inflammation). The usual route is via eye drops, but oral and intravenous means of treatment are sometimes necessary.

Due to potential side effects and potential improper use, topical corticosteroids are seldom prescribed by non-eye doctors. The most common unintended side effect is elevation of the intraocular tension, suggesting glaucoma. Those whose pressures go up are "steroid responders," estimated as 10 percent of the general population. If the pressures go down after discontinuation of the steroid drops, then the patient can be followed as a glaucoma suspect, along with usual tests to confirm the absence of glaucoma. However, if a steroid responder, a patient needs to be followed as a potential patient for glaucoma.

Newer corticosteroids of lower potential risk relatively to causing glaucoma, are available, such as Lotemax (Alrex). Combinations of antibiotics and steroids are common, such as Blephamide (sulfa and steroid), Tobradex (tobrex and steroid), and now Zylet (tobrex and alrex). The combinations with lower "risk" steroids using alrex as the steroid lowers the potential rise in intraocular pressure down to 2 percent. Not all who get a steroid pressure response would get glaucoma.

Another potential undesirable side effect of topical steroids is the tendency to make treatment of early Herpes Simplex (HSV) corneal infection more difficult, and since it is difficult even for eye doctors to differentiate pink eye from HSV, this is the main reason primary care doctors are warned not to use steroid eye drops. Cataracts can be caused potentially, but most steroid cataracts are a result of long-term oral use of steroids.

Cyclosporin (Restasis)

Cyclosporin (Restasis) has an anti-inflammatory reaction when used topically for keratoconjunctivitis sicca (dry eyes), with a potential of stimulating normal tear production. Supplement lubricants are also needed, especially at early stages. Used systemically, this medication is used in nonocular problems involving immunosuppression.

Nonsteroid Anti-inflammatory Drugs (NSAIDs)

NSAIDs are used more frequently now as a substitute for corticosteroids, especially pre and postoperatively for cataracts (Ocufen and Voltaren), and for pain relief and allergy (Acular).

Antiallergy Agents

Over-the-Counter (OTC) Eye Drops

OTC eye drops are available without a prescription and make up the majority of such medications, containing vasoconstrictors such as Visine (take the red out), or combined with antihistamines as in Visine A, Naphcon A, and Opcon A. Care must be taken with such medications to avoid overuse as will be reflected in rebound redness of the eyes. Typically the effect seems to wear off faster, and a person puts more drops in to form a cycle, whereby rebound vasodilatation occurs, similar to the overuse of nose drops.

Prescription Allergy Eye Drops

Prescription allergy eye drops are naturally more expensive and can include corticosteroids. Mast cell stabilizers take longer for an effect but may have a more lasting influence, such as Crolom, Zaditen, and Alomide. Combination-effect medications add antihistamines and other means of prolonged effect, and can give more immediate relief. These include Optivar, Zaditor, Alocril, and Patanol. Prolonged use may be necessary. Steroids are, of course, better, but must be limited in regard to long-term use.

Lubricants (Artificial Tears)

All artificial tears are OTC, or nonprescription. Most are intended to be used intermittently or on a schedule of up to four times a day, or more. Conditions such as air travel or exposure to air conditioning or heat in an automobile may require additional usage. Some lubricants are thicker to last longer. Some are in ointment form for use at bedtime.

Preservative-free artificial tears are less likely to be irritating (some people are bothered by the preservative used in artificial tears), but are more expensive due to the individual packaging involved. It is literally all right to try artificial tears if the eye feels irritated. They basically do no harm, unless used, along with other eye drops, more than eight times daily, and may give temporary relief to a minor condition requiring no more treatment. It they don't help, then seeing an eye doctor may be indicated. Those with truly dry eyes probably should have a regular schedule of use, not just put a drop in the eye once in a while when it gets real bad.

Contact lens wearers, including soft contact lenses, can have their ability to use the contact lenses, full time, limited by dry eyes, and there are special lubricating drops to use with soft contact lenses, which should be in the contact lens section for solutions at the drug store. Lasik can cause dry eyes, either transiently postoperatively or continuously.

Some artificial tears available OTC include Bion Tears, Genteel, Hypotears, Moisture Eyes, Refresh, Soothe, Systane, Tears Naturale, Theratears, Visine Tears, and store brand lubricants.

Glaucoma Eye Medications

Cholinergic Agents

Cholinergic agents, most commonly pilocarpine, make the pupil small, and are used primarily in treating narrow-angle glaucoma, potential narrow-angle glaucoma, or mixed glaucoma (part open angle and part narrow angle). Because of the small pupil, dark adaptation is diminished, but on the positive side there may be less dependency on glasses.

Adreneric Agents

Adreneric agents are the opposite of cholinergic agents but also improve drainage of the intraocular fluid from the eye. Common medications of this type are Propine and Alphagan P. Such drops are seldom used as the primary means of treatment, but can be of great use as an add-on medication to another glaucomatous treatment.

Beta-Blocker Eye Drops

Beta-blocker eye drops are quite effective and have been approved as a first line of treatment. Timolol, for example, is available as a generic drug, and can be used once or twice daily with good results. Disadvantages include a needed warning to those with asthma or emphysema, who may note a worsening of symptoms on beta blockers, including those with chronic cough or heart conditions (usually a low heart rate). If a patient is already taking beta blockers for hypertension or heart disease, the eye drop form may not be so effective for the treatment of glaucoma. Examples of beta blockers are Timolol (Timopic, Betimol, or Istalol), Levobulonol (Betagan), or Betoxalol (Betoptic-S).

Carbonic Anhydrous Inhibitors

Carbonic anhydrous inhibitors can be used topically, having been long available as oral medications, such as Diamox. Orally, Diamox is useful for acute situations requiring rapid decrease of intraocular pressure, but due to side effects chronic use is not advisable. In eye drop form, such as with Trusopt or Azopt, this type of medication can be a good add-on for the treatment of glaucoma. The combination with a beta blocker called Cosopt, has been successful, though requiring use two or three times daily for full dosage.

Prostaglandins

Prostaglandins are the newest and most promoted eye drop treatment for glaucoma, and work by aiding better drainage of fluid from the eye. They can be a primary medication, with the advantage of use only once daily, usually at bedtime. Combinations with beta blockers are being developed. Disadvantages include expense, since none are generic. Examples include Xalatan, Lumigan,Travatan, and Rescula. Side effects include possible darkening of eye color and growth of eyelashes.

Over the Counter Eye Drops (OTC)

There are a great number of eye drops available without a prescription. Some are all right to use, and others are pure "snake oil." For example, Similasan makes a drop for "cataract care" and describes its use as relieving symptoms of diagnosed cataracts and aging eyes. The "take the red out" drops, such as Visine, are all right for occasional use, but cause rebound redness if used too often. Visine actually makes multiple eye drops now, for vasoconstriction to take the red out, to anti-allergy drops such as Visine-A, and plain lubrication artificial tear drops. It is because of the old-time Visine, to take the red out, that warnings have been made relative to overuse.

Artificial tears are available in multiple brand names and basically are all right to use for any suspicious indication of irritation. Minor irritants are soothed even if one does not have truly dry eyes. It should be pointed out that some eye drops may be irritating to the eyes, including artificial tears, if a person is sensitive to the preservative in the drops, usually BAK, or benzylkonium chloride. Preservative-free artificial tears are available, but the packaging makes them more expensive.

Boric acid drops were often used, why, I don't know. Another old-time OTC medication was Argyrol, containing silver. This remedy ceased being useful years ago, but acted as an astringent, resulting in burning, reflex tearing, and actual destruction of the mucous glands of the conjunctiva. Though the drops caused irritation, the patient sometimes felt that the eyes felt better after the irritation ceased. Once I had a patient who was "hooked" on Argyrol and could not be pacified by the fact that this drug was no longer available. He had argyrosis of the conjunctiva, causing a grey look to the white of the eye. Since he couldn't get Argyrol anymore, he was putting mercurochrome into the eye to give a comparable burning effect.

Contact lens solutions are available, and patients usually follow recommendations of their eye doctor. Special artificial tears are acceptable for use while wearing contact lenses. Then there are special solutions for cleaning and maintaining the contact lenses, all available OTC.

WHO PAYS AND HOW

Years ago, there was a simple answer to who pays for medical care: it was the patient, and usually cash on the barrel head. Certainly that was true for eye care, even after health insurance became common. The arrival of Medicare changed things a lot, but instead of the expected demise of medicine, it has become the standard by which medical payments are measured. The usual and customary fees are now rarely paid in full, paradoxically only by those who have no insurance. However, the "sticker price," though necessary for bookkeeping, is rarely paid for medical services.

In the development of union benefits, eye care became involved. In addition to medical care, and dental care, eye care was desired as a work benefit not taxable to the employee. This idea spread to many industries, including schools and government jobs. Included benefits were typically the ability to have an annual eye exam for all members of the employee's family, plus glasses every one or two years. Contact lenses could be covered, or at least an allotment used for the purchase of new or replacement contact lenses. These plans have been good for the patients and eye doctors, but perhaps over utilized. For example, one may be inclined to get another pair of glasses this year to take advantage of the benefits, even if one already has one or more satisfactory pair of glasses. And average people cannot afford to have everyone in the family to have their eyes examined every year.

Then, when retired, or of Medicare age, a person naturally feels that these eye care benefits should continue to be available. For sure, for health reasons it would be good, since the elderly age group needs to be conscientious about getting their its eyes examined due to the increased likelihood of age-related eye disease. However, Medicare does not pay for "routine" examinations, and the comprehensive eye examination is considered routine. Medicare will pay for an eye examination if there is a diagnosis, such as cataracts or glaucoma suspect, but the portion for measuring the vision, the "refraction," is not covered. This is because Medicare looks at this part of the exam as just for someone wanting a new pair of glasses, and does not recognize that a diagnosis of eye disease, or the severity, cannot be measured without measuring vision. Therefore, the Medicare patient with cataracts or other eye problem is charged a carve-out fee for the "refraction." This is difficult for patients to understand, for good reason.

Health maintenance organizations (HMOs) have provided a solution. Most of these health plans do include coverage for eye examinations, and sometimes glasses, as part of a senior plan. Medications can also be included to a degree. However, in these plans, a patient is limited to the selection of a doctor from those available in the HMO, and no longer has control of their Medicare benefits. The eye doctor also would have to be on the HMO-approved list.

Medicaid patients usually do have eye care coverage. An eye examination may be covered for yearly or every-other-year comprehensive examination. Glasses may also be a benefit, but restricted to every two years or longer, along with evidence of change of prescription. Among the problems, however, is the fact that not all doctors, including eye doctors, will accept Medicaid patients, because of the very low fees provided. There are only a few designated optical shops that can accept Medicaid glasses prescriptions.

Health benefits, including surgery, are covered by Medicare, HMOs, General Insurance, or Medicaid. Medicare usually controls the acceptable fee, Part A for the hospital fee and Part B for the physician fee. For example, if a usual and customary doctor's fee is $2,000, Medicare may, for example, only recognize $800 as acceptable, and then pay only 80 percent of $800, or $640. A secondary insurance would then do likewise: recognize only the $800 fee, and then pay the 20 percent not paid by Medicare, $160. HMOs pay their participants even less on the Medicare dollar, and then, of course, Medicaid pays much less yet. Though this may sound unfair, and doctors think so, they are bound to accept these fees in full payment. The recent exception, as mentioned, is in "presbyopia surgery." The example given is fairly close to representing what has happened to compensation for cataract surgery via Medicare. I refer to our "sticker price" when discussing "usual and customary" fees, because no one intends to pay it. However, if doctors lower their "sticker price" in an attempt to help lower costs of health care, then Medicare would only lower the compensation further. Occasionally, patients who consider themselves financially in need, and who do not have any secondary insurance, will ask the doctor to accept the Medicare payment as payment in full. Unfortunately, the doctor is bound by Medicare rules to not to accept the Medicare payment as payment in full, and is obligated to bill the patient for the 20 percent owed.

20

EYE CARE–THE WAY IT WAS AND THE WAY IT WILL BE

ORIGIN OF THE OPHTHALMOLOGIST

Who knows who was the first caveman eye doctor. Certainly eye diseases date back to antiquity, such as infectious and contagious trachoma, which was even recently the most common disease in the entire world. Treatments of eye diseases are described in Egyptian, Greek, Roman, and Arabic artifacts. Early treatments were sometimes rather gross, for example, couching of cataracts. This practice, originated in India, amounted to using a sharp stick to penetrate the cornea, and push a dense cataract back into the vitreous so as to unblock the pupil to allow some vision.

According to Dr. Fred Blodi, my mentor at the University of Iowa, couching of cataracts was the procedure of choice for 2,000 years, spreading from India to the Western world. It was performed by traveling barbers, since true medical surgeons felt it beneath their dignity. An incisional approach was introduced in 1750 by Dr. Daviel, but the complication rate was so high that couching continued until around 1800, when Von Graefe perfected a better incisional approach.

Cataract surgery progressed to the use of sharp knives to make an incision in the upper cornea, large enough to push out the cataractous lens from behind the pupil, per Von Graefe. By this time spectacles became available to improve vision. Postoperative care, however, amounted to extreme limitation of activity to allow the wound to heal. Enforced bed rest with sand bags on each side of the head was necessary for weeks. Postoperative activity improved with the use of sutures.

Suturing of wounds was not available for eye surgery until very tiny, curved, and sharp needles were developed, so as to avoid distortion of eye tissue during the suturing process. Suture material was silk initially, and this was well tolerated by the eye, but the sutures had to be removed later, and this was often difficult. Absorbable sutures are usually too irritating to eye tissues, but in recent years, microfine nylon sutures are used and these eventually fade away. Most recently, in cataract surgery; no sutures are usually necessary due to the tiny self-sealing entry wounds. As you may imagine, postoperative activity following cataract surgery is now minimally limited.

Anesthesia for cataract surgery has varied according to availability and need. Early general anesthesia was too often involved with ether and similar nauseating agents, such that the procedure could be made painless, but the complications from vomiting often greatly also complicated the visual results. Later a combination of a big dose of Demerol, something like Valium, some local injection of an anesthetic, and eye drops was used to get through the procedure with good results. More recently, the services of an anesthesiologist are utilized, incorporating medications that make a patient not only pain free but amnesic and cooperative during the outpatient surgery.

Hospitalization of a cataract patient in the 1950s was usually for four to five days, to make sure the patient was all right to return home. Sometimes, since the other eye was also usually ready for surgery, the second cataract was also removed, resulting in only a bit longer hospitalization. In the 1970s a trend for outpatient surgery for cataract patients was initiated by ophthalmologists, and this soon became the preferred routine. It was not long before Medicare insisted on only outpatient cataract surgery, as if it was their idea in the first place. One advantage of outpatient surgery is that on the first day following surgery, a patient is examined in the office, and a much better evaluation of an early result is possible than at a hospital bedside.

Then a renowned ophthalmologist invented another "stick" to put into the eye to remove the cataract. Dr. Charles Kelman invented the phacoemulsifier, sometimes confused with a laser, but actually an ultrasound technique for breaking up the cataractous lens and sucking it out (aspiration). This allowed a tiny incision through which the "phaco" tip could be inserted, often not requiring suturing of the wound. Results for the neophite ophthalmologist were initially either really good or really bad. This was because of swelling of the cornea, which was common for beginners in the technique, something usually just temporary. Skills with this technique since the 1970s have resulted in increased excellence in results and in less operative time.

Then the intraocular lens implant made a comeback in cataract surgery. The intraocular lens implant was a great innovative idea, but early lenses were poorly manufactured, and the insertion of these lenses often meant loss of the eye. Later, in the late 1970s, improved IOLs became the newest and best alternative in cataract surgery. To not require the thick aphakik glasses, and the ability to predict the outcome such that the power of the IOL may result in less need for glasses than preoperatively, meant this was the newest and greatest innovation in cataract surgery. However, insertion of these lenses required a larger incision, requiring sutures, and there developed a decrease in enthusiasm for the microincision involved with phacoemulsification (PKE).

Along the way, it became necessary for an ophthalmic surgeon to become familiar with the operating microscope. Prior to this, eye surgeons used what are called "loupes," magnifying lenses worn either as an addition to the front of a regular pair of glasses, or without glasses. These loupes magnified images only a little bit, perhaps 50 percent, but were greatly helpful in cataract surgery, and all other eye surgeries. Other fields of surgery have adopted the use of loupes, but not nearly enough by my observation. The use of a microscope is difficult at first. It is like looking at some fingers working, without the assurance that they are your fingers, and watching any mistakes literally magnified. Eventually experience has allowed the confidence that this is the very best way to do cataract surgery. An assistant was literally required in the learning phase, to ensure that visualization of the operative field was not too limited. Medicare eventually declined payment for an assistant in cataract surgery, but by then we were generally able to do without an assistant. This is also a trend for all surgery, as far as Medicare denying assistant surgery payment, meaning often that a surgeon better have a really good scrub nurse.

So after going back to a larger sutured cataract incision to insert optically well polished and manufactured intraocular lens implants, foldable IOLs evolved. The acceptance of these innovations was mixed at first. There were those quite anxious to return to the microincision involved with phacoemulsification (PKE), but it was true that the optics of the foldable IOLs was not as good as the rigid IOLs. Eventually, however, the quality of the foldable IOLs improved, such that an argument about better vision with the rigid IOLs no longer was valid. As a result, the great majority of cataract surgery now involves foldable IOLs. And, of course, with foldable IOLs came the resurgence of phacoemulsification PKE. This continues to be the method of choice in cataract removal, in spite of the introduction of new techniques involving actual laser or special irrigating techniques.

The latest innovation is the accommodative IOL. This is a boon for the cataract patient in order to see well without glasses. However, current models are not perfect, and require an adaptation process from the "brain," perhaps not totally predictable. These lenses are in the manner of either multifocal, or lenses that react much like original accommodation (focusing). The newness of these IOLs makes it likely that there will be newer and better lenses in the future. All of this is changing so fast that it makes the head of an ophthalmologist swim of an ophthalmologist in practice, like myself, during the last few decades.

The practice of ophthalmology is not all cataract surgery, for sure. In fact, it has been difficult for those in authority, like my superiors in the U.S. Air Force, to categorize my services as either "surgical" or "outpatient." A general ophthalmologist is certainly one who spends more time in the office than the operating room, and is proud to have it that way.

The old eye doctors were actually EENT, or Eye, Ear, Nose, and Throat, doctors. Theirs was among the first specialties in medicine, established in 1896. Training as pure ophthalmologists began in the 1930s and 1940s, but the Academy of Ophthalmology and Otolaryngology continued to have combined meetings and certificates until 1979. Many of the old EENT doctors were forced to pick one or the other specialty in their later years of practice, eye or ear, nose, and throat.

To be an ophthalmologist requires from three or four years of specialty training beyond medical school and internship. Such training more or less qualifies an ophthalmologist to perform all phases of treatment and surgery. Naturally, some ophthalmologists were inclined to be interested in certain phases, and eventually fellowships resulted by means of preceptorship (working with a doctor who specialized in certain treatments) or extended residency (an extra phase of learning provided by a department of ophthalmology affiliated with a medical school). Certainly with the explosion of technology it has become impossible to be an expert in all phases of ophthalmology.

Among the subspecialties in ophthalmology are vitreoretinal, pediatric, corneal and external disease, neuro-glaucoma, ophthalmic pathology, and ophthalmic plastic surgery. Those who do not subspecialize are called general ophthalmologists. At first, since this applied to me, I felt like I was being likened to a general practitioner (GP), like I was not a specialist. Later, knowing what experiences I have had, I have felt like this is just what I am, a general ophthalmologist, and am proud of it. Many subspecialists have a problem existing outside an academic environment. However, further subspecialization seems to be a predictable trend in the future.

THE ORIGIN OF AN OPTOMETRIST

In the meantime, optometry has undergone tremendous change also. Spectacles were developed in the thirteenth century. For centuries, tradesmen sold spectacles, often like a traveling salesman. Bifocals appeared in the twentieth century. Some opticians later became more specialized and referred to themselves as refractive opticians, following learned techniques of measuring and correcting visual defects. The term optometrist was adopted in 1904, meaning "one who measures optics."

My father was an optometrist, trained at the Illinois College of Optometry in the 1930s. He was an "ethical" optometrist and required to be so as a member of the Iowa State Optometry Association. This meant that he could not advertise other than put his name and profession in the newspaper or phone book, no advertising of any special deals, etc. My uncle, also an Iowa optometrist, was criticized for becoming employed by Sears and forming an optical shop there. Subsequently, as result, his membership in the state optometry association was in jeopardy. Eventually, advertising among optometrists became necessary, especially when chain optical shops appeared, which were also eventually able to employ optometrists.

My father did not charge for an eye examination, his financial reward being in the glasses he prescribed and dispensed. However, it was a given that a recommended pair of eyeglasses would be the result of all of his examinations. Fees for an optometric eye examination became a routine about the time that Medicare entered the picture. Also, contact lenses arrived in the 1960s.

If the profession was in trouble, as some predicted, the arrival of corneal contact lenses revived and energized the field of optometry. Optometrists became specialists in contact lens fitting, whereas ophthalmologists were slow to embrace this means of treatment into their practices. Emboldened by success, and for business reasons, organized optometry pressed for more privileges, first with diagnostic pharmaceutical agents (DPAs). This allowed the use of topical anesthetic eye drops, for example, for use in testing for glaucoma with intraocular pressure measurement. Also involved were dilating drops and cycloplegic drops for examination advantage via a large pupil. Prior to that time, one way of differentiating between an ophthalmologist and optometrist was whether you had your eyes dilated during the exam.

Later, encouraged by the results of influencing state legislatures, organized optometry pushed for therapeutic pharmaceutical agents (TPAs). Since the scope of practice of optometrists, like such as chiropractors and podiatrists, is determined in most states by the state legislature, it has been more necessary to convince a legislator than a medical control board as to the qualifications to expand the scope of practice for optometry. While admittedly organized ophthalmology recognized problems potential to such expansion to TPAs for optometry, it became not a matter of debate or common sense, but rather a battle of political manipulation, and the optometry organizations seemed better at this.

As result, optometrists have been granted therapeutic privileges of various degree, depending on the state involved. In some states, the treatment of glaucoma is allowed, with many or most of the available topical eye drop medications permitted. In other states, a more restrictive use of medications for glaucoma and other limitations may be encountered. The main problem, other than granting such privileges in general, is that the treatment and prescribing principles vary per state.

INTERACTION OF OPHTHALMOLOGY AND OPTOMETRY

So the roles of ophthalmologists and optometrists have changed through the years, and the need for cooperation seems obvious. Ophthalmologists need help in providing necessary eye care, and the answer does not mean providing more ophthalmologists. The answer involves better use of optometrists in coordination with ophthalmologists. The answer also does not, I believe, lie in the attempt to make an optometrist the equal of an ophthalmologist.

Admittedly there is a turf war between optometry and ophthalmology. This is not secret, as it was mentioned in the September issue of the *U.S. News and Report*, under the subject of paramedical influence on the practice of medicine. Organized optometry is threatening doing eye surgery, with state approval, and naturally this has organized ophthalmology very upset. This is because it is so totally ridiculous. Where would the optometrist who has not become a medical doctor learn to do surgery? Who would insure such a person? Part of the encouragement may be in regard to laser surgery, since it now has become possible to perform a lasik operation without any surgical (use of a cutting knife) intervention. The laser can create the corneal flap and then complete the procedure. Some might not call this really surgery, but those optometrists who look forward to this loophole into the practice of ophthalmology may be naive in thinking that it is easy. Then there is question about the laser and lasik manufacturing companies and their roles in encouraging optometrists along these lines.

What seems to work best is the cooperation of ophthalmologists and optometrists in the same office. Under these circumstances, the true value and expertise of an optometrist in eye care can be best utilized. Some ophthalmologists, for political or other reasons, have utilized ophthalmic technicians in office care of patients. These technicians can be of great help, and are trained with the help of the Academy of Ophthalmology, but are not of the same value in practice as an optometrist. Because of training, an optometrist can be of use in screening new patients for pathology, and can be given responsibilities in the absence of the ophthalmologist far beyond that which should be delegated to a technician.

This brings up the subject of training of general doctors and their assistants. Years ago, medical school training was fairly universal in the Unites States. Everyone had basically the same curriculum. The first two years were basic sciences, during which nonclinical physician instructors seemed to do their best to flunk out medical students. The last two years were the clinical years, during which rotation to various specialty services took place. Eventually, family practice became one of these fields. Ophthalmology lectures were commonly given in a basic degree, and a rotation through the ophthalmology department was an option.

More recently, trends in medical school training have encouraged early declaration as to the expected final intent as far as the type of practice a student plans. This assumes, of course, that such students have some insight into what they want before having a taste, so to speak, of what is available. Along the way, different schools apparently modified their curriculum such that it was less predictable as to the final result (general education) upon graduation. Ophthalmology, as a subject, was usually not routinely covered, even in minor detail. The result, is that medical doctors know very little about the eye. This book, for example, is meant for them as much as for the general public.

Following medical school is the internship. A rotating internship was the rule, meaning that, like in medical school, a broad experience was obtained in treating patients for all manners of problems during this year, from delivering babies to working in the emergency room. Along with the changes in medical curricula, it has become routine to replace the rotating internship with a more specialized one. For example, if you intend to become a surgeon, you may rotate through anesthesia and surgical subspecialties (a la the TV show "Gray's Anatomy"), but not any nonsurgical fields. A potential ophthalmologist would spend much of the year in the ophthalmology department, trying to qualify for a residency, if not already accepted.

The end result has been that the newer MDs know even less about the eyes than former doctors. Nevertheless, general physicians in HMOs are often placed in a screening gatekeeper role, with the responsibility to treat minor eye problems if possible, and limit referrals to an ophthalmologist unless necessary. In the meantime, through need, the emergency room specialty physicians have become actually better in diagnosing and treating eye disease, within limits.

Current trends in medicine have involved medical assistants to an increasing degree. Nurse practitioners obtain a masters degree, and are allowed to treat patients, with or without supervision of a medical doctor. Physician assistants work with doctors in varying levels, sometimes able to examine, treat, and prescribe. Neither of these groups is able to help in eye care to the degree of an optometrist, whose training is usually in excess of even the general physician in the ability to recognize, treat, and determine the additional need for treatment by an ophthalmologist.

What is needed, is not to encourage optometrists to compete with ophthalmologists, but the potential of better cooperation within the two groups. The potential for involvement in eye care can be beyond even the wildest dreams of optometrists, but only in cooperation with ophthalmologists who can better train them to be effective.

There will be doubters as to whether such cooperation is possible, like my optometrist father, who died with Alzheimer's a few years ago. In perhaps my last conversation with him at his care facility, I told him that I was working on a way for optometrists and ophthalmologists to better get along. In one of his rare cogent moments, he said "That will be the day."

THE WAY THINGS CAN BE (AS I SEE IT)

There are likely changes to be expected in the provision of ophthalmic care. The trend to subspecialization is likely to continue. The role of the general ophthalmologist will change also. High-volume cataract surgeons will probably make the general ophthalmologist less interested in performing cataract surgery. They will still have plenty to do managing glaucoma, macular degeneration, and other diseases. The generalist may accept a referral role in cataract surgery, sending the patient off for surgery and resuming care postoperatively.

I also can foresee a trend for subspecialists to combine general ophthalmology care with their subspecialty, since it is often difficult in a nonacademic environment to practice a pure specialty. It is also possible that there will be more combinations of subspecialties, such as pediatric and neuroophthalmology.

A new subspecialty I can predict will be cataract and refractive surgery, combined. The way things are going, the cataract surgeon, and especially the presbyopia surgeon, is expected to provide a near perfect result, starting with distance vision. This implies the need for touchup or revision surgery, a la lasik, to eliminate residual refractive error (usually astigmatism) as something expected and included in the surgical fee. Currently, most lasik surgeons have given up other types of ophthalmic surgery, including cataract surgery. The traditional cataract surgeon is not one who has usually spent much time with other refractive surgery such as lasik. The new comprehensive refractive surgeon will be required to do lamellar and surface corneal surgery plus lens procedures, such as cataract and clear lens extractions.

The optometry role has great potential for change. I think all optometric schools should be associated with a medical school ophthalmology program. The basic optometry course can be similar to what it is now and the graduate able to practice optometry along the lines of the traditional need in providing refractive and contact lens care, being a doctor of optometry (OD). However, the curriculum can be supplemented by lectures and clinical inclusion of patients with eye disease, as provided by the ophthalmology department. A complementary role with ophthalmology can be experienced such that the role of the optometrist can be better utilized.

The issue of comanagement by optometrists of cataract and refractive surgery patients can be better resolved if ophthalmologists are involved in the training of optometrists. The potential of large-volume surgeons increasingly dominating the field, and general ophthalmologists withdrawing from cataract surgery, means that the referral role of optometrists will be even greater. Also there will be then increased responsibility of postoperative care, not expected to be provided by the large-volume surgeon, comanagement.

It also should be possible for an optometrist to spend extra time under clinical training in the ophthalmology department. More detailed and concentrated training can be provided in such diseases as glaucoma and external eye disease. If an optometrist is to assume responsibility of treatment of such things as glaucoma, as now allowed in many states, it is best that the optometrist know as much as possible about glaucoma. Included in the learning process will be the realization that such treatment decisions are by no means simple and uncomplicated, so as to recognize the need for extra training and insight as to when to ask for help. Such extra training will not be so as to further confuse the difference between an optometrist and an ophthalmologist, but to actually emphasize the difference. Such an optometrist could be designated as an MOD, or a medical optometrist.

I realize that in order to make such changes, there would have to agreement to cooperate by organized optometry and ophthalmology, something many believe impossible. It would have to be a national change. The optometrists could still be licensed by each state, but the scope of practice would have to be universal throughout the country. And certain schools could not call their graduates MODs unless they had completed the prescribed courses by their associated ophthalmology department. (It is noted that some dental schools, in parts of the country, call their graduates doctors of dental medicine [DMDs], as if to imply that they are more medically trained than a doctor of dental surgery [DDS].)

And no, the OD or the MOD will not be doing surgery. If they want to do surgery, they can go to medical school. However, this can be made to be a more viable option. After completing optometry school training, a graduate can be offered the opportunity to go to medical school to complete just the last two years, graduating as an MD. The assumption, of course, is that such a person will want to become an ophthalmologist for an additional three or more years training, and internship can be added to this. It is conceivable that the ophthalmology department may be influential in helping the optometry student be accepted for this abbreviated medical school experience, and imply the likelihood of being accepted into the ophthalmology resident program. It can be noted that osteopathic physicians have parallel, but not the same, education as in a medical school, and are doctors of osteopathy (DOs) rather than MDs. Yet osteopathic school graduates can be accepted into any ophthalmology residency and become general or subspecialized ophthalmologists.

Is this unfair, to allow a shortcut to becoming an MD? Well currently, it becomes necessary for an optometry graduate to go four more years to become an MD. The first two years are spent in basic sciences as usual. Though the optometry school basic sciences are not the equivalent of medical school, they could be improved with medical school guidance. Also I think credit should be given for the time spent in optometry school, including patient contact not experienced by beginning medical school students. And, as far as fairness is concerned, I think this opportunity to shorten medical school training to two years should be also extended to dentists and nurse practitioners. They also have basic science and medical background, and may decide along the way that they would like to be an M.D.

Dentists have shown interest in general health and medicine, hoping to incorporate such knowledge in the treatment of their patients. Some are perhaps practicing medicine more than intended. I have heard that some dentists even perform blepharoplasties. Oral surgeons have become part of medical practice for many years. Their residency programs have taken place parallel to medical school programs, and their ability to treat surgically in the head and neck areas has been remarkable, considering that they have not gone to medical school. They also can do blepharoplasties, I understand. I am not saying that oral surgeons should be required to go to medical school, but it is natural to assume that if they did, they would be better prepared for the work that they do. Of course, graduates of a medical school would not be forced into a particular area of treatment if they, for example, wanted to become family practitioners or other specialists. Pre-dental school, I understand, as far as requirements is similar to pre-optometry. Basic sciences and general medical background are also part of dental school, and I think similar credit should be allowed so that a dental school graduate can finish medical school in two years.

Nursing school and pre-nursing, of course, are parallel, in some degree, to that of medical school. Many nursing schools now provide a graduate degree so as become a nurse practitioner, someone who is considered trained to be able to practice medicine alone, without a physician supervisor. The graduate program, I believe, is three years. Why not offer a nurse practitioner who is interested in medicine to an advanced degree the opportunity to become a medical doctor by finishing medical school in two years? Actually, I am told, this opportunity is already offered. It makes sense to me, but then I have digressed.

Back to eye care. The future is very bright for eye care. Note the explosion of technology for the treatment of cataracts, presbyopia surgery, new medications for glaucoma and macular degeneration, and talk of medication to bring back optical nerve function. The delivery of eye care will be expertly delivered by both ophthalmologists and optometrists. Just wait and *see.*

I recently attended a lecture by Professor James Walter (Loyola Marymount University) on bioethics, and he pointed out that the greatest changes in the history of medicine have occurred in the last twenty-five years. My personal experiences have certainly supported this fact. Also he described the evolution of doctor perception from being the paternalistic and trusted advisor for health care in the 1950s, to being a that of technician under the employ of the patient for personal benefit in the 1960s, to being, in the 1970s and beyond, an entrepreneur or vendor in providing commodities for personal use. I guess I, as a physician, am shocked at this characterization, but I can certainly agree with a drastic change during the forty-four years as a practicing ophthalmologist. Now that I am semiretired, I can observe and sympathize with both the doctor and the patient point of view. However, if patients are to be making decisions for themselves in eye care, then they need to be well informed so as to make intelligent decisions. I am writing this book to help people know the basics about their own eyes, to point out some of their choices in eye care, and to help them make informed decisions.

GLOSSARY

abrasion. A scratch. *See also* **corneal abrasion.**

accommodation (uh-kah-muh-day-shun). Increase in optical power by the eye in order to bring things into focus when closer.

acuity. Clarity. *See also* **visual acuity.**

after cataract, secondary cataract. Remnants of the lens in the eye following extra-capsular cataract extraction (now routine) that may become enlarged and opacified so as to obstruct vision again.

age-related macular degeneration (AMD, ARMD) (mak-yu-lur). A retinal disease that becomes more common with increased age, and affects the central or reading vision because of degenerative effects on the macular part of the retina.

amblyopia (am-blee-oh-pee-uh), **"lazy eye."** Incompletely developed vision, usually in one eye, present without anatomical evidence of a problem, but due to various causes.

Amsler grid (AM-slur). A test card with lines formed in a grid formation such that distortion suggests central vision problem, as with macular degeneration.

anterior chamber angle. The fluid-filled space inside the eye between the iris and the cornea, important in determining difference between open- and narrow-angle glaucoma.

aphakia (ay-fay-kee-uh). The state of the eye after the normal lens has been removed, as in cataract extraction.

aqueous (ay-kwee-us), **aqueous humor.** Clear waterlike fluid that fills and nourishes the interior of the front part of the eye. Normal amounts maintain the proper intraocular pressure of the eye, but excessive amounts lead to increased intraocular pressure and glaucoma.

astigmatism (uh-stig-muh-tiz-um). An out-of-round condition, whereby the cornea is not perfectly spherical like a basketball, but somewhat of the shape of a football (in exaggeration). Resultant imperfect focus affects vision at all distances.

atrophy (ah-trophy). A loss of function due to withering away of substance.

basal cell carcinoma. A type of skin cancer.

Bell's palsy. Paralysis of muscles innervated by the seventh cranial nerve, resulting in problems closing the eye, raising the brow or mouth.

benign (bee-nine). Noncancerous.

bifocals. Eyeglasses that usually have distance vision correction in the top, separated from near vision correction in the bottom of the lens.

binocular vision. A cooperative result of both eyes working together in somewhat equal degree, resulting in a stage of depth perception.

black eye (ecchymosis). A collection of blood under the skin from injuries near the eye, but not necessarily involving the eyeball itself.

blepharitis (blef-uh-ri-tus). Inflammation of the eyelid margins.

blepharoplasty. Surgery to reduce excess skin of the eyelids.

blepharospasm (blef-uh-ro-spaz-um). Spontaneous, unpredictable closure of the eyelids, resulting in increased blinking or inability to keep the eyelids open.

blind spot. A normal sightless area within the visual field representing where the optic nerve enters the eye and not usually evident because of the ability of the brain to mask the defect. *See also* **visual field test.**

blowout fracture. A fracture of the orbital floor that can involve periorbital tissues (fat, nerves, and muscles), usually caused by blunt trauma.

botox (botulinum toxin). An injectable medicine with powers to temporarily paralyze or weaken muscles; used to treat blepharospasm, but also to reduce wrinkles and headaches.

brow lift. A surgical raising of the eyebrow tissue due to sagging effect on ability to open the eye.

canthus (can-thus). The angle formed by the junction of the upper and lower eyelids, lateral toward the ear and inner toward the nose.

capsular bag. The cellophane-like bag of tissue that encloses the normal lens of the eye, which is left in place in modern surgery so as to form an envelope into which the intraocular lens implant may be placed. If becomes opacified, it is called a secondary cataract, something cured by YAG laser capsulotony.

cataract. Opacification of the normal lens of the eye, resulting in blurred vision and corrected by removal of the clouded lens, called cataract extraction. Usual cause is advanced age, but also trauma, diabetes, or medication.

cellophane maculopathy (epiretinal membrane, macular pucker, preretinal fibrosis). A thin layer of scar tissue that affects good macular vision, like macular degeneration, but which may respond to observation or surgery involving peeling away the membrane.

central retinal artery. The first branch of the ophthalmic artery that supplies most of the retina.

central retinal vein. Correspondingly the main vein exiting the eye via the optic nerve.

central serous retinopathy. A syndrome involving swelling of the macula.

central vision. The most sensitive vision from the macula, used in reading.

chalazian (sha-lay-zee-un). Inflamed cystic swelling of a meibomian gland.

choroid (kor-oyd). A layer made up mainly of blood vessels between the retina and sclera.

ciliary body. The part of the uvea extending from the iris that controls focusing and forms intraocular fluid (aqueous).

color blindness. Limited ability to determine shades of colors, usually hereditary.

cone. Color- and form-sensitive retinal receptor centralized in the macula.

congenital. Condition present at birth.

conjunctiva (con-junk-tie-vuh). Transparent mucous membrane covering the outer surface of the eyeball, except for the cornea, and lining the inner surface of the eyelids.

conjunctivitis (con-junk-tee-vi-tis), "pink eye." Inflammation of the conjunctiva; infectious, viral or bacterial, mechanical or allergic.

convergence. The coordinated movement of the eyes inward, toward each other, to follow an object as it becomes closer.

convergence insufficiency. A coordination problem affecting the ability to maintain binocular vision when viewing an object as it becomes closer, as in reading.

cornea (kor-nee-uh). The windowlike clear bubble of tissue covering the iris through which light is transmitted through the pupil to focus onto the back of the eye (retina).

corneal abrasion. A scratch of the cornea involving loss of surface epithelial layer cells.

corneal transplant. A surgical procedure involving replacing most of a diseased cornea with a healthy donor cornea.

corneal ulcer. An infection of the cornea involving deeper layers.

cranial nerve. One of twelve nerves coming directly from the brain and serving areas of the head and neck above those affected by spinal nerves.

crossed eyes. *See* **esotropia**.

cryotherapy. *See* **freezing treatment**.

cycloplegic refraction (si-kloh-plee-jik). Examination of the eye involving cycloplegic eye drops capable of relaxing the ability of the pupil to become smaller and temporarily paralyzing the focusing muscles.

cystoid macular edema. A fluid buildup affecting the macula, sometimes after cataract surgery.

dacryocystitis. Infection of the tear duct system between the eye and the nasal cavity.

dacryocystorhinostomy (DCR). Creating a new opening from the tear duct to the nose.

diabetic retinopathy (ret-in-ahp-uh-thee). Development of typical hemorrhages, exudates, and sometimes new blood vessels complicating long-term and late-stage involvement from diabetes mellitus (disease of abnormal blood sugar regulation).

dilated pupil. Enlargement of the pupil from natural iris muscular action or artificially as result of drugs, injury, or medications.

diopter (di-ahp-tur). A refractive term describing optics in metric form.

diplopia. *See* **double vision**.

drusen (dru-zin). White spots deep in the retina, which when present in the macula may indicate early signs of age-related macular degeneration.

dry eye syndrome. Insufficiency of lubricating tears of the eye that causes irritation. If severe in involvement of the cornea, it is called keratoconjunctivitis sicca and if accompanying rheumatoid arthritis, called Sjögren's syndrome.

dyslexia (dis-lek-see-uh). A neurological problem affecting reading, not due to eye disease, and usually permanently resistent to treatment.

ectropian (ek-troh-pee-un). An outward turning or falling away of the eyelid from the eyeball, usually of the lower lid.

edema (ih-deem-a). Swelling due to fluid accumulation.

emmetropia (em-uh-troh-pee-uh). The refractive state of little or no imperfection of distance vision without effort, like a camera set for focus to infinity.

endothelium (end-o-thee-lee-um). The specialized single-cell layer lining the inner surface of the cornea, of critical need for nutrition and regulation of water content.

endophthalmitis. An infection within the eyeball, and therefore serious.

entropian (en-tro-pee-un). The turning inward of the lid margin and lashes toward the eyeball, usually of the lower lid, and related to tissue laxity.

epicanthus (ep-ee-can-thus) **epicanthal fold.** Vertical skin fold common in infants of all races, which diminishes with facial development, except in Asians, whereas it continues to some degree into adult age. The common cause of pseudostrabismus, looking cross-eyed when not.

epiretinal membrane (cellophane retinopathy, macular pucker, preretinal fibrosis). A thin sheet of scarlike tissue that can effect macular vision.

episclera. A layer of connective tissue separating the conjunctiva from the sclera, when inflamed, called episcleritis.

epithelium (ep-ih-thee-lee-um). Outermost layer of tissue covering the cornea, conjunctiva, and skin of the eyelids.

esotropia (ee-soh-troh-pee-uh), **cross-eyed.** Deviation of one eye toward the nose, can be intermittent or constant.

excimer laser. A cold laser used in refractive surgery to shape the cornea.

exotropia (eks-oh-troh-pee-uh), **wall-eyed.** Deviation of one eye laterally, toward the ear.

extraocular muscles (eks-truh-ahk-yu-lar). Six muscles that move the eye in coordinated fashion (lateral and medial rectus, superior and inferior rectus, plus superior and inferior oblique muscles).

eyelid margin. The edge of the eyelid where eyelashes grow.

eyelids. Skin-covered structures that protect the eyes and regulate vision by controlling the amount of light exposed to the eyes. Lubricating tear flow is distributed by blinking.

eye socket (orbit). The roomlike space in the head occupied by the eyeball and adjacent tissues.

facial palsy. *See* **Bell's Palsy**.

farsighted. *See* **hyperopia**.

floater. A visible spot, of various shapes and sizes, which moves with movement of the eye, but is usually not large enough to diminish vision. Onset is usually spontaneous. When accompanied by light flashes, it is important to have a good examination by an eye doctor, to be sure the floaters are only a minor nuisance and not a sign of retinal detachment.

fluorescein angiogram (flor-uh-seen). After the dye fluorescein is injected into a vein, photographs of the retina blood vessels are taken for diagnostic purposes.

fovea (foh-vee-uh). The most sensitive center of the macula, made up entirely of cone cells.

fundus. The most posterior part of the retina visible with an ophthalmoscope.

fusion. The blending of images performed by the brain so as to provide binocularity and depth perception.

giant papillary conjunctivitis (GPC). An allergic form of conjunctivitis usually associated with protein deposits on soft contact lenses, and largely eliminated by use of daily wear disposable soft contact lenses.

glaucoma (glaw-koh-muh). A common, sight-threatening disease of the optic nerve that is usually associated with elevated intraocular pressure beyond the tolerance of the optic nerve.

gonioscopy (goh-nee-ahs-koh-pee). Examination of the anterior chamber angle, where aqueous fluid drains from the eye, by means of a special contact lens optical instrument called a goniolens.

Grave's disease. A form of hyperthyroidism involving inflammatory changes of periocular tissues and telltale signs involving the eyes.

herpes simplex (cold sore virus). A virus that causes an infection of the cornea, which can be stubborn to treat and recurrent.

herpes zoster (shingles). A virus which that attacks skin areas along nerve fibers, causes blisters that can be painful, and which can involve the eye when the ophthalmic division of the facial nerve is effected. Treatment of eye complications can be prolonged.

histoplasmosis (hiss-toh-plaz-moh-sus). A fungus infection which that may cause a delayed reactive swelling and visual effect years later.

hordeolum (stye). A pimplelike infection involving the eyelid.

hyperopia (hi-pur-oh-pee-uh), **farsightedness.** A focusing imperfection such that, unlike with emmetropia where the eye is already in focus for distance, the eye must use its accommodative powers to bring things into focus, and then even more, of course, to bring things into focus at near. Glasses or contact lenses can correct the need for extra focusing.

hypertension. High blood pressure.

hypertensive retinopathy. Special retinal hemorrhages caused by hypertension.

hyperthyroidism. Overactivity of the thyroid gland, which can cause eye complications.

hypertropia. One eye higher than the other eye in alignment.

hyphema (hi-fee-muh). Blood in the anterior chamber, the space in front of the pupil and iris, usually caused by blunt trauma.

hypotony. Low intraocular pressure, usually an unhealthy sign.

intraocular lens (IOL). An artificial lens placed inside the eye in addition to, or to replace, the normal lens of the eye.

iris. Pigmented tissue, the colored part of the eye, behind the cornea and which that forms the pupil. Pupil size is controlled by iris muscles.

iritis. Inflammation of the iris tissue, which is very common as a complication to any injury to the cornea, or surgery, but which can occur spontaneously without apparent cause.

keratitis. Inflammation of the cornea.

keratitis sicca. *See* **dry eye syndrome**.

keratoconus (kehr-uh-toh-koh-nus). Degenerative corneal steepening and astigmatism.

keratome (kehr-ah-tome). An instrument for shaving a thin flap in the cornea.

keratometry. Measuring the corneal curvature by means of a keratometer.

keratoplasty. Surgery on the cornea. A corneal transplant is called a penetrating keratoplasty.

laceration. A cutting or tearing type wound.

lacrimal duct, tear duct. The tubular connection including the lacrimal sac, from the eyelid to the nasal cavity for drainage of tears.

lacrimal gland. A tear-producing gland located in the upper outer part of the orbit.

laser. A high-energy light source that cuts, burns, or destroys tissues, and which that can be used for various purposes in eye treatments, as well as treatments elsewhere in the body.

lasik (lay-sik), **laser in situ keratomileusis.** A laser procedure involving a corneal flap for treatment of refractive errors such as myopia, astigmatism, and hyperopia.

lazy eye. *See* **amblyopia**.

legal blindness. Status when the better eye cannot see better than 20/200, even with correction, or has reduction of visual field to 20 degrees or less.

lens. The natural lens of the eye.

leukocoria. A white pupil, usually caused by advanced cataract.

limbus. The junction of the cornea with the sclera, the outer edge of the cornea.

low vision. Term used for quite poor vision, less then 20/200, and often requiring special visual aids.

macula (mak-yu-luh). The central area of the retina, the focal point for reading and color vision.

macular edema. Swelling of the macula.

macular hole. A hole in the macula which effects vision, different from holes causing retinal detachment.

magnetic resonance imaging (MRI). A special radiologic technique.

malignant. Potentially destructive, as in cancerous.

melanoma. A tumor involving pigmented cells. The most common eye malignancy.

metastatic. A tumor which that has spread to another part of the body from original site.

migraine. A special headache syndrome which that can have other neurological signs.

multiple sclerosis (MS). A neurologic disease that often has eye involvement.

myopia (mi-oh-pee-uh), **nearsightedness.** A condition whereby distance vision is blurred and the eye is in focus at some point nearer than infinity, often as if the eye is too large. A corrective minus lens can bring distance objects into focus.

nearsightedness. *See* **myopia.**

neovascularization (nee-oh-vas-kyu-lur-ih-zay-shun). Growth of abnormal new blood vessels, usually involving the retina or iris, which can be a complication of diabetes retinopathy, closure of the central retinal vein, or macular degeneration (wet kind).

neuro-ophthalmologist. An ophthalmologist with special training in neurological diseases, with attention to how the eyes can be involved and improved.

nevus (mole). A pigmented lesion which that can also be found in the eyelids, conjunctiva, iris, or retina.

nystagmus (ni-stag-mus). A jerky movement of the eyes, intermittent or constant, hereditary or acquired, usually involuntary, and potentially a problem for vision.

occipital lobe. The part of the brain located in the back of the head where vision is processed.

ocular prosthesis (artificial eye). Used to replace an absent eye.

oculoplastic surgery. A subspecialty in ophthalmology concerned with cosmetic and functional aspects of the tissues around the eyeball.

ophthalmoscope (ahf-thal-muh-skohp). Instrument for visualizing the interior of the eye via the pupil, especially the posterior pole of the retina.

optic disc, optic nerve head. The optic nerve visualized from the interior of the eye, containing nerve fibers and blood vessels.

optic nerve. The second cranial nerve, carrying sensory nerve fibers from the retina to the brain.

optic neuritis. Inflammation of the optic nerve. *See also* **multiple sclerosis.**

orbit (eye socket). The bony room in which the eyeball is located; part of the skull.

orbital cellulitis. Infection of the orbit.

pachymetry. A technique for measuring the thickness of the cornea.

pan retinal laser photocoagulation (PRP). A technique with laser to treat retinal neovascularization.

papilledema. Swelling of the optic nerve as evidenced by appearance in fundus exam, usually related to increased cerebrospinal fluid pressure, and to be differentiated from papillitis (swelling due to inflammation).

patching. Covering one eye, either in therapy for corneal injury, or to encourage the nonfavored amblyopic to develop better vision.

perimetry (puh-rim-ih-tree). A test, usually automated, for determining the field of vision of an eye; used most commonly in glaucoma testing and for neurologic deficit.

peripheral iridotomy. A surgical or laser procedure to create an extra hole in the iris, other than the pupil, for treatment or prevention of complications such as glaucoma.

peripheral vision. Side vision, or travel vision as compared with central or reading vision.

phacoemulsification (fay-koh-ee-mul-sih-fih-kay-shun). The revolutionary procedure introduced by Dr. Charles Kelman, making microincision stitchless cataract surgery the procedure of choice, using ultrasound waves to break up the lens material.

photodynamic therapy (PDT). A special laser procedure for treatment of certain types of wet macular degeneration.

photophobia (foh-toh-foh-bee-uh). Excessive sensitivity to light, a symptom of iritis.

pingueculum (pin-gwek-yu-lum). A yellowish thickening of the conjunctiva near the cornea, associated with increased vascularity.

pink eye. *See* **conjunctivitis.**

posterior capsular opacity (secondary cataract). The clouding of the intact posterior portion of the capsular membrane left in place in cataract surgery.

posterior chamber. The space inside the eye between the back of the iris and the vitreous gel, occupied normally by the lens, and into which a posterior chamber intraocular lens is placed.

presbyopia (pres-bee-oh-pee-uh). Age-related loss of focusing (accommodation) due to loss of elasticity of the lens, affecting everyone; usually evident by age forty-five.

presbyopia surgery. A surgical approach to loss of focusing ability, available either at the time of cataract surgery or with clear lens extraction, and utilizing an accommodative IOL or multifocal IOL. Also can involve surgery or laser treatment of the cornea or ciliary body.

progressive addition lens (PAL). A multifocal spectacle lens that gradually changes correction from distance correction to reading correction, without a line as seen with a traditional bifocal. It has features of a trifocal, but is not a true trifocal.

proliferative retinopathy. A severe form of new vessel formation sometimes complicating diabetes.

pseudotumor cerebri. A disease involving increased cerebrospinal fluid pressure, of unknown cause, and one cause of papilledema.

pterygium (tur-ih-gee-um). A wedge-shaped growth of conjunctiva extending onto the cornea, which, if large enough, can threaten to block the pupil and require surgery.

ptosis (toh-sis). Drooping of the upper eyelid which that is usually surgically correctible. May actually be complicated by drooping of the eyebrow, called brow ptosis.

pupil. The round opening in the iris that controls light entering the eye, like the aperture of a camera.

recurrent corneal erosion. A spontaneous or postinjury problem whereby the surface epithelial cells of the cornea flake off and expose the cornea to painful irritation, repeatedly, until final proper healing occurs.

refract. To optically bend or change direction of light rays.

refraction. Testing a person's eyes for visual imperfection, and possible need for glasses, or other alternatives.

refractive error. Optical defect effecting vision due to hyperopia, myopia, astigmatism, or presbyopia, usually expressed in metric form by diopters, as in a glasses prescription.

refractive surgery. Surgical or laser procedures performed to improve on the uncorrected level of vision of the eyes.

retina (ret-ih-nuh). The thin layer of nerve tissue lining the back two-thirds of the eye, like wallpaper, and which is the light-sensitive nerve tissue directing image impulses to the brain via the optic nerve.

retinal detachment. Separation of the retina from underlying tissues, like wallpaper peeling off the wall. This is a medical emergency because delayed repair may result in permanent loss of part or all vision in the eye.

retinoscope (ret-in-oh-skohp). An instrument allowing the user to objectively estimate with fair accuracy the refractive error of the eye. It is especially important in examinations of children or poorly responsive patients.

rod. Light sensitive cells which that allow appreciation of vision at low light levels, resulting in night vision.

Schirmer test. A measure of tear function, involving placement of a filter paper strip inside the lower eyelid.

Schlemm's canal (shlemz). A channel for drainage of aqueous fluid via the anterior chamber angle trabecular filtering system into the blood stream.

sclera (skleh-ruh). The white of the eye, which is a dense, protective white covering over the deeper sensitive ciliary body and retina, from the cornea to the optic nerve.

scleral buckling. A surgical technique for treatment of retinal detachments popularized by Dr. Charles Schepens, with usual good success, and often resulting in a myopic shift in refractive error.

scleritis. Inflammation of the sclera, usually painful; sometimes cause unknown.

scotoma (skuh-toh-muh). A blind spot in the vision, which may be normal in the case of the optic nerve entrance, but may be the early sign of glaucoma.

shingles. *See* **herpes zoster.**

slit lamp. An illuminating microscope that allows examination of the front part of the eye in great detail, routine use of which gives an eye doctor great advantage.

Snellen chart. The standard chart for measuring visual acuity.

squamous cell carcinoma. A type of skin cancer which also may involve eyelids.

squint. *See* **strabismus.**

stereopsis (stehr-ee-ahp-sis). Binocular depth perception.

steroid. Short for corticosteroid, an anti-inflammatory drug. Also sometimes used to refer to androgenic steroid, in sports reference.

strabismus (struh-biz-mus). Eye misalignment, such as being cross-eyed.

stroke. A sudden lack of blood supply leading to damage, as in the brain. A similar situation occurs in the eye, an extension of the brain, with retinal artery or vein occlusion.

sty (hordeolum). A pimplelike infection of the eyelid, usually due to staphylococcus.

subconjunctival hemorrhage. A usually spontaneous and insignificant bleeding into the conjunctiva, which causes concern due to a red eye.

tarrsorrhaphy (tar-soar-ah-phee). Surgical sewing the eyelids together, as may be needed for temporary protection of the eye in facial nerve palsy.

temporal arteritis (giant cell arteritis). An inflammatory disease of blood vessels that can involve the eye, as well as the brain.

tonometry (tuh-nah-mih-tree). Measurement of intraocular pressure.

toric lens. A lens that corrects astigmatism, such as in a contact lens or intraocular lens implant.

toxoplasmosis (tahks-oh-plaz-moh-sus). An unusual infection which that also may involve the eye as a retinochoroidal inflammation with resultant typical scar formation.

trabecular meshwork (truh-bek-yu-lur). The filtering meshwork type tissue that filters and regulates the flow of aqueous fluid from the eye via the anterior chamber angle.

trabeculectomy. A glaucoma surgical procedure involving increasing the drainage via the trabecular meshwork area.

20/20. The standard of normal visual acuity, meaning one can see at 20 feet what one should see at 20 feet. *See also* **Snellen chart.**

uvea, uveal tract (yu-vee-uh), uveal tract. A vascular pigmented layer which that extends from the iris to include the ciliary body and then the choroid in the rear of the eye.

uveitis. Inflammation of the uveal tract, anterior when iritis and ciliary body, and posterior when involving the choroid.

verteporfin (Visudyne). A specific dye used in photodynamic therapy.

visual acuity. Measurement of ability of the eye to see, and recorded such as 20/20 if normal, or 20/200 or worse if legally blind.

visual field. A dimensional measurement of the central and peripheral vision.

vitrectomy. A surgical procedure for removing the vitreous gel from the eye.

vitreous (vit-ree-us). The optically clear gel which that fills the cavity between the lens and the retina.

vitreous detachment. A separation of the vitreous gel from the retinal surface, which causes symptoms such as floaters and light flashes, at least temporarily, but usually causes no problems. However, sometimes it leads to a retinal hole, leading to a retinal detachment, and therefore a thorough eye examination is indicated.

wall-eyed. *See* **exotropia.**

YAG laser. A special laser that can be focused, for example, in use to perform an iridotomy in glaucoma treatment, or capsulotomy in the case of clouding of the posterior capsule following cataract surgery (secondary cataract).

zonules (zahn-yoolz). Suspensory fibers from the ciliary body that support the lens and are involved in accommodation.

INDEX

About the Author

CLYDE K. KITCHEN, M.D., is a member of the Senior Active Staff of St. Jude Hospital, Department of Ophthalmology, in Fullerton, California. He is an Ophthalmologist in practice for more than 36 years.